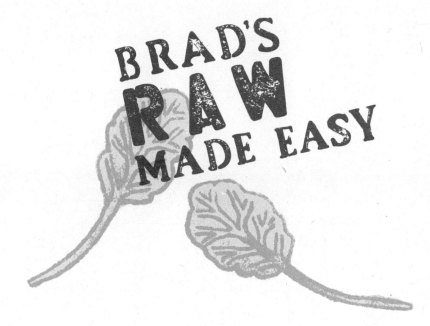

BRAD'S RAW MADE EASY

BRAD'S RAW MADE EASY

The Fast, Delicious Way to
Lose Weight, Optimize Health, and
Live Mostly in the Raw

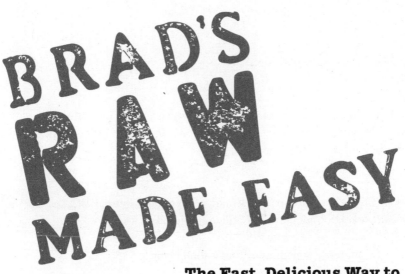

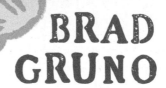

BRAD
GRUNO

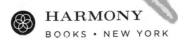

HARMONY
BOOKS · NEW YORK

Published in the United States by Harmony Books, an imprint of the
Crown Publishing Group, a division of Random House LLC, New York,
a Penguin Random House Company.
www.crownpublishing.com

Harmony Books is a registered trademark of Random House, LLC, and the
Circle colophon is a trademark of Random House, Inc.

Library of Congress Cataloging-in-Publication Data
Gruno, Brad.
Brad's raw made easy: The fast, delicious way to lose weight, optimize health,
and live mostly in the raw/Brad Gruno.—First edition.
pages   cm
1. Reducing diet—Recipes. 2. Raw food diet—Recipes. 3. Weight loss.
I. Title. II. Title. Raw book.
RM237.5G78 2014
613.2'65—dc23   2013020205

ISBN 978-0-385-34812-6
eBook ISBN 978-0-385-34813-3

Printed in the United States of America

Book design by Lauren Dong
Interior photographs courtesy of Natasha Shapiro, Allison Davis, Jeff Skeirik,
    Pam Gruno, and Alex Mack
Chart on pages 204–205: © Environmental Working Group, www.ewg.org.
    Reprinted with permission.
Insert photographs copyright © 2013 by Ellen Silverman
Jacket design by Jess Morphew

10 9 8 7 6 5 4 3 2 1

First Edition

To my daughter, Eva—here's to a very healthy
second chapter of our lives together

Contents

Introduction

Not many people are grateful for the economic dot-com crash of 2001. When the economy tanked I lost everything I had—but it turned out to be the best thing that ever happened to me. It brought me, in the most roundabout way possible more than a decade ago, to the raw food that literally saved my life.

I grew up in Bucks County, Pennsylvania. My family ate a typical American diet of meat and potatoes (steamed kale—what's that?), and a lot of them smoked and drank and never exercised. I left home when I was twenty and moved to California to work as a plumber with my uncle. There I met my now ex-wife. After we were married we decided to move to Pittsburgh so I could begin working with her father in his strip-mining business.

Several years later, I got divorced and moved to Atlanta to work with my father in the telecommunications industry. After learning how to run crews and operations from my father-in-law and honing my business management skills with my father, I built up the confidence to go out on my own. A tremendous amount of money was being poured into the fiber optics construction industry, and I eventually became successful with my own business. I had houses and a yacht and fancy friends in fancy places. I thought I had it made.

That's when the dot-com industry crashed. All the investors pulled out, with no intention of ever paying the outstanding million-dollar invoices, and my $30 million company went down the tubes. I'm not kidding when I say it happened overnight. And believe me, when everything gets torn out from under you, you find out who your friends are really quickly.

There I was with no prospects, no money, no home, and no ideas about what to do next. I did not have the college education that might have opened certain doors for me, but I had the entrepreneurial spirit I had learned from my father. So I called my aunt and uncle and asked them if I could stay for a while. They said of course, and I moved back home to Bucks County, where they welcomed me with open arms and let me stay in an apartment in their barn. Not surprisingly, I became depressed. I moped around the apartment, eating a lot of junk; I weighed a good forty pounds more than I do now. Gradually I got bored with wallowing in self-pity and started asking myself what I could do. I took a good look in the mirror and thought, "You know what? You might not have had control over what's happened already, but the one thing you can control is how you take care of yourself. You can control what you eat and you can control how you move." So I started going to the gym.

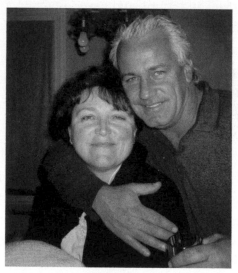

Brad Before

My wonderful aunt Joyce was always health conscious and liked to go to a raw food restaurant, Arnold's Way, located in nearby Lansdale, Pennsylvania. It's a popular place, and owner Arnold Kauffman (who will play an important role in this story) is known and respected for his knowledge about raw food, his kindness, and his willingness to educate people who want to learn more about a raw food lifestyle. When

Aunt Joyce saw that Arnold was offering a raw food preparation class, she was thrilled and signed right up. After a few sessions, she invited some of my cousins over for a five-course, all-raw ("raw" means un-cooked, or heated to no more than 115°F) meal, including appetizers, a main course, and dessert. It was incredibly delicious. A few days later I watched a documentary called *Eating* on a DVD my aunt had in the house. In it, different physicians discuss what a diet high in processed foods and low in fruits and vegetables does to the human body and how eating a non-plant-based diet can contribute to heart disease, dia-betes, and other illnesses. The message of the film inspired me, and the next day I went 100 percent raw.

Let me just say that I would never suggest that anyone go raw cold turkey, no matter how well prepared you think you might be! My body rebelled, big time. For the first three weeks my life was hell. I had flu-like symptoms. I had massive headaches and no energy. I could barely get out of bed, even though I dragged myself to the gym and tried to work out. My face was even breaking out. I was a wreck!

Because my aunt Joyce had stacks of books about nutrition and health lying around the house, and I'd read them all, I was mentally prepared for what can happen during a food detox. The residue of those decades of junk food and steak dinners and red wine and white bread and mashed potatoes and heavy desserts that left me so stuffed I could barely get up was getting purged from my body. When the headaches hit or the aches and pains got intolerable, I would just grit my teeth and go with it. I knew that feeling bad was temporary. I had to ride it out and stop myself from scarfing down a burger or cooked food in an effort to make me feel better in the short term.

When I'd been raw for about three weeks, Aunt Joyce took a look at me and smiled. "Brad," she said, "you are just starting to glow. Your skin—it's incredible! Go take a look if you don't believe me."

I took a look, and she was right. My acne had disappeared. My eyes were clear. It was as if the proverbial light at the end of the tunnel was shining on me. I have to admit I was kind of shocked at how good I looked. Not only that—I was starting to feel really good, too.

Now I was more determined than ever to stick to a raw food

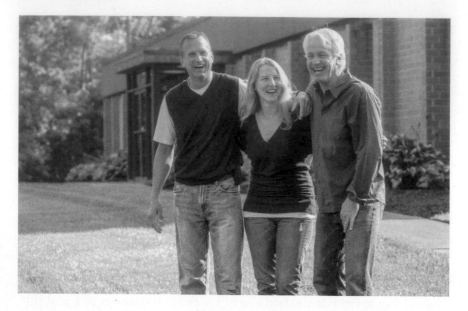

lifestyle. I didn't want to cheat, or slow the process down. There was no way I was going back to my old life and my old bad habits.

I ended up staying completely raw for more than a year. I even gave up the red wine I loved. Once those initial three weeks of misery had passed and my energy level started to ratchet up, I went to the gym nearly every day. I worked out hard, because I knew it was important to sweat it out—to get those toxins out of my body every way I could.

I didn't notice the weight falling off in the first couple of weeks, but I am not kidding when I say I lost several pounds each day. It was incredibly exciting to step on the scale. The more I'd sweat, the better I'd feel. I was determined to keep going.

It was almost like I was on a mission. I'd tried plenty of exercise plans and diets before, but they'd never worked (and I'd never been able to stick to them, either) or made me feel this good. It took only three months for me to lose forty pounds and get back to the same build that I'd had when I was twenty-one (size 31 jeans—hallelujah!).

But it wasn't just about the weight and how my body had transformed from pudge to ripped. I was working on the inside, too. I took up yoga and learned how to meditate. I went on a retreat, where I sat with myself, without talking or looking at anyone else, for ten days, just meditating. I had the luxury of time to look at everything in my life and bluntly evaluate my past. It was tough, but it was also exhilarating. I realized that almost hitting bottom was the wake-up call I'd needed. I was nearly fifty years old, and thanks to good raw food and good rigorous exercise and taking a good hard look at my hopes and dreams, I'd never felt or looked better in my life.

There was, however, one thing that I'd had a tough time with when I went raw: the crunch factor.

In the first three months on my raw diet, I ate very simply. Every morning I'd get up before dawn and go to the gym, and then I'd come back and make a whole pitcher of green smoothies. That would keep me going until noon. Every three days I'd go to the grocery store and come back with eight or nine large bags brimful of fresh fruit and veggies and nuts and seeds. I'd wash everything, cut it up, mix it all together, and then divvy it up into plastic containers that I stacked neatly in the fridge.

I'd eat two of these salads a day. I knew I had to do this because when you're hungry, you look to what's there already to assuage your stomach rumblings. I knew myself—if my gorgeous salads were already cut up and packed up and waiting for me, and if I'd premixed

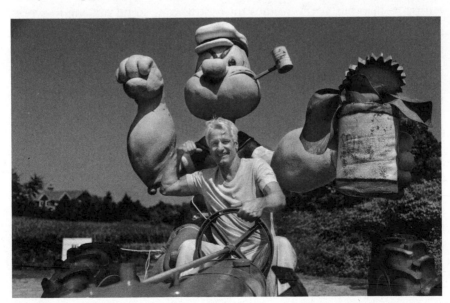

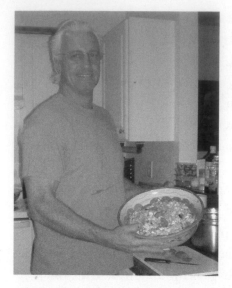

the ingredients for a raw dressing made from cashews, red bell peppers, and sunflower seeds (see Brad's House Dressing in chapter 8), I'd make a smart choice.

The only thing missing was the crunch. Sure, crisp red peppers and cucumbers had a satisfying bite to them, but they weren't enough. When I was driving somewhere I wanted to be able to reach in the back of the seat and find something to munch on. This is where Arnold comes back into the story. I hung out in his restaurant with other raw foodies who had more experience than I did and could talk to me about how I was eating. It was my first experience with a community that was bonded together by its love for a certain type of food, and it was deeply satisfying for me to be around such cool, interesting, educated, and helpful people.

Because I wasn't working at the time, I told Arnold that I'd be happy to help out at the restaurant in any way, so he put me to work peeling bananas for his famous banana whips. I was a silent observer to how graciously Arnold helped all the customers who came to him for food and for advice about their health or weight issues, or preparing raw food.

One day, as I was making a batch of Arnold's bread (flaxseeds for beneficial omega-3 fatty acids, buckwheat groats for protein, carrots and other vegetables and spices for fiber, micronutrients, and taste—it was just as satisfying as a yeast-and-flour bread used to be for me), it dawned on me that I could use a dehydrator, a machine that slowly removes moisture from food, to make vegetable chips that I could put into a bag and carry with me whenever I felt the need for a crunchy snack.

I put a few bunches of kale in the food processor with some buckwheat groats and flaxseeds, pulsed it up, and dehydrated the mix overnight. When I sampled it in the morning I couldn't believe how delicious it was. I experimented, adding other vegetables such as carrots, bell peppers, scallions, and garlic to make the chips even more satisfying and nutritious—it was almost like having a meal in a bag. After the vegetable chips were created, I went on to experimenting with crunchy kale chips, which have become my most popular item. I never dreamed that my chip would become a business. I just made them because I missed having something to munch on!

Fast-forward two years and I was still living in Bucks County, still living the raw foods lifestyle, still practicing yoga and going to the gym. I worked construction to pay the bills, but I was ready for the next phase of my life, whatever that would be. I started attending Go Green conventions, figuring that my construction background might be useful in the green arena. At a show in Philadelphia I was talking to exhibitors about solar energy and putting up solar panels, when I saw the Zukay Live Foods booth advertising raw salsa. The man selling the salsa, Scott Gryzbek, had a big bowl full of regular tortilla chips to dip in the salsa for sampling. I went over to talk to him and said, "Why would you have that unhealthy chip with that beautiful salsa? You need raw chips." Scott laughed and said he hadn't yet found a chip he liked. I told him I made my own chips and he said he'd love to try them. We exchanged numbers and about a month later I met him at a trade show. He absolutely loved the chips. So did his employees, and all the people who came to sample his salsa flipped out for them, too. He said, "You know what? You might have something better than I have here."

Did it dawn on me that, even though I was eating raw and loving my raw chips, I would end up selling raw food? No, it did not!

I jumped at the opportunity to join Scott at an upcoming Go Green convention in New York City. He'd sell his salsa and I'd help him set up the booth and put out my chips for sampling. I'd had the dehydrator running for days making what I thought would be enough chips.

Well, the show opened up at 11 a.m., and as people came in and out I stayed in the background. I was enjoying watching Scott work the crowd, but practically every time someone dipped one of my chips into the bowl, they'd say, "Oh, wow, this is delicious. What's up with this chip?" Scott would point at me and tell them to talk to the guy in the back. Much to my surprise, the more I talked, the more comfortable I felt explaining how I made the chips. I glanced over to the salsa table and saw the chips rapidly disappearing, which floored me. After an hour of being surrounded by visitors, Scott pulled me aside and said, "Look, I'm sorry but you've got to take these chips off the table because nobody's looking at my salsa!"

That was the precise moment when the big lightbulb switched on in my head.

As I drove back home my mind was racing. By a total fluke I had made a raw snack that tasted good and was really good for you. Not many crunchy products can make those claims. But I also knew that my chips would not be an inexpensive food to produce and package. Who, I wondered, would want to buy a bag of darn small chips for seven bucks in an economy where so many people were struggling to pay their bills?

There was only one way for me to find out. I contacted my good friend Jerry Fritz of Linden Hill Gardens, who ran the weekly Ottsville Farmers' Market. Jerry always has been a huge supporter of mine, so I thought, what better place to try out my chips?

I set up a table, and before the market had even fully opened everybody was buying my chips. I sold out before noon. The people who stopped to sample and buy were incredibly interested in the chips, not just because they tasted so good, but because, they explained, it was important for them to find the most nutritious food possible so they could feel good and take the best care of their families.

I told them that these chips were real food, and not full of additives. They weren't made from potatoes or cornmeal but from real vegetables and seeds and other good things. And they weren't fried or baked, but dehydrated below 115°F, the magic number needed to preserve all the nutrients and the enzymes of the ingredients. The more these customers learned, the more they wanted to buy.

At this point I knew I needed some expert advice in the food industry. Fortunately for me, Steve McDonnell, who is a really nice guy and owns the organic food company Applegate Farms, lived right up the road. He hooked me up with Dana Sinkler and Alex Dzieduszycki, the two guys who started the now hugely successful Terra Chips brand in their one-car garage in New York City. They understood my vision, and the more I talked to those in the know in the food business, the more I realized that I had found something that wasn't just good for me but was good for everyone. I had finally found my passion, and my authentic self.

I knew I needed to continue to learn while developing my business, so I started going to events hosted by prominent raw food speaker and educator David Wolfe. I also looked at his Longevity Warehouse website and learned what kind of products he sold and what customers were responding to. I felt energized every time I left one his events.

I was determined to grow my business slowly and do it right, so for months I continued to work at local farmers' markets, learning more about organic foods and farming. I volunteered to help my neighbors Dan and Rose Nagel of Swallow Hill Farm plant and harvest if they'd teach me more about growing food organically. This incredibly generous couple told me to use their single-car garage as a dehydration room. I got it all set up and pretty soon I had about forty dehydrators going on full-blast, all day long, making chips.

My sister, Pam, came up with the name "Brad's Raw Foods" and designed the packaging. I now had enough inventory to supply several local health food stores. My brother-in-law, Richard Finch, provided my first investment to get up and running. Being in these stores gave me enough confidence to start knocking on the door of Whole Foods. Let's just say I was persistent—all I wanted was to get my chips into one Whole Foods store. Just one! My persistence paid off; I got the news a buyer at Whole Foods was going to take a chance on me. Hearing that was one of the best days of my life! Brad's Raw Chips were going to be sold in the Whole Food stores on South Street in Philadelphia and in Princeton, New Jersey.

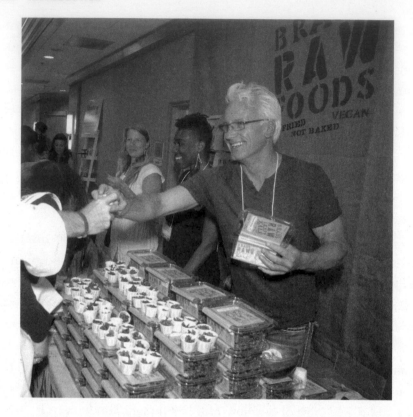

I loved passing out samples in the stores. Even in Whole Foods, which has an educated clientele, many people didn't know very much about raw foods. I told folks how going raw had saved my life and gave me my health and career back.

I couldn't wait to get in that store and tell people about my chips. In fact, I would get there at 9 a.m. when I didn't need to be there till 11, and I'd stay until the store was practically ready to close—that's how inspired and revved up I was. It was thrilling to see people's faces light up when they sampled my chips. Often these customers didn't even know what kale was. Many were just learning the benefits of healthy eating and were thrilled to find a healthy, crunchy snack, especially if they had been skeptics. Usually, a sample was all they needed—and then they were converted. Seeing someone embrace this kind of food and then become more interested in a raw food lifestyle was deeply satisfying.

Before I could catch my breath, I was selling more than $14,000 worth of chips per month in one store. Whole Foods took notice and told me I was going to be in thirty-eight more stores. Thirty-eight? How was I going to supply them when I could barely keep up with the orders in one store? Luckily, Whole Foods really believed in me and granted me a loan through their local producer loan program, which enables small businesses like mine to continue to grow. That money allowed us to move into a larger facility. As I look back, I honestly can't believe this business, which started in a one-car garage, is now a $25 million dollar company. I have to pinch myself sometimes!

I called my business partner and good friend from my old telecommunication days, Walt Gruger, and together we built a proprietary dehydration system that cut our production time in half. I was able to expand my team and hire experienced salespeople to get my chips into more and more stores. One of the first was Jaime Cahalan. We literally went from store to store on the East Coast, talking and giving out samples all day long. There were so many people who were curious about raw food and better nutrition but had no idea what eating raw means, or how to implement it into a more healthy lifestyle. And this is when I first began seriously thinking about writing a book.

What I hope to do with *Brad's Raw Made Easy* is to demystify and simplify what it means to eat raw food. It truly doesn't have to be hard. I'll show you how eating raw really means adding more of, not taking away from. Arnold Kauffman would say, "I'm not telling you to take anything away from your diet. I just want you to eat more. Eat more fruit, eat more salads." By doing so, you'll gradually shift your eating away from entirely cooked to healthier, more raw foods. Start out with a good green smoothie in the morning, and you'll see how much more energy you have.

Believe me, I'm the last person who'd ever say, "You need to be 100 percent raw in order to reap the benefits of this lifestyle." That's too hard for most people to swallow (literally!), and that goes for me, too. Eating 80 percent raw and 20 percent cooked is the right balance. If I want a steak once in a while, I'm going to eat one, and I'm going to enjoy it.

I hope you will see this book as one part of the whole that is the raw food community. I never thought of myself as someone who changed other people's lives. Then one day, when I was in the P Street Whole Foods store in Washington, D.C., stacking the chips that I had just delivered, the assistant grocery manager Mansur Aman said, "You know, Brad, you're like the pioneer of raw food."

I was stunned. "You've got to be kidding," I said.

"No, you really are," he insisted. "Your chips opened up the whole raw section to other raw items. If that's not a pioneer, I don't know what is!"

On my amazing journey to raw, I found my purpose in life. I went through some hard times, but a lot of people helped me and believed in me and my ideas, and as a result I learned how to believe in myself and take a bit of risk to create what I was sure would work. I look back at what I once had and I wouldn't exchange it for the wonderful, passion-driven, healthy, and fun-filled life I have now for anything. My goal is to build the biggest and the best raw food company and help people all over the world improve their diet and their health.

Let raw do for you what it did for me!

PART I
THE RAW TRUTHS

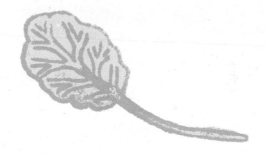

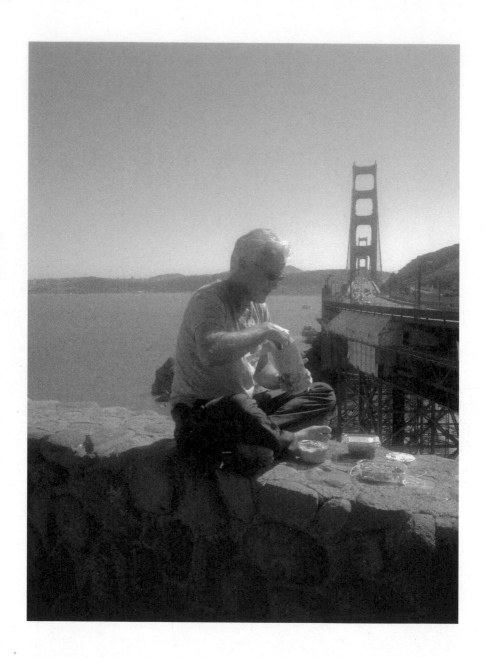

1
THE SCIENCE BEHIND A RAW FOODS DIET

What could be more invigorating than a meandering walk in a verdant park on a bright sunny day? Think of breathing in the sweet, fresh air and feeling the spring of the grass beneath your feet. Think of how all your senses would be delighted, giving you mental clarity and a deep sense of connection to the physical world. Think of how just plain good you'd feel.

That's how you would feel if your diet consisted of only fresh, delicious, nutrient-rich food from nature. That's what happens when you eat raw foods. So how do you add more of these foods without breaking the bank or working in the kitchen all day? Keep reading.

WHAT IS RAW FOOD?

A raw foods diet is one that consists of raw fruits, vegetables, nuts, seeds, sprouts (including grains and legumes), root vegetables and squashes, fresh herbs, spices, fermented foods, and seaweeds. These foods are never heated beyond 115°F, which is why you will hear many people in the raw food community refer to this as eating only "living foods."

It is a myth to think of a raw foods diet as one of deprivation, where you can eat only "rabbit food" such as lettuce and carrots! There are countless satisfying dishes that can be created by following the raw food guidelines. Nearly anything that you loved in your old cooked diet can be created uncooked for your eating pleasure.

NUTRITIONAL INFORMATION YOU NEED TO KNOW ABOUT EATING RAW

What makes a raw foods diet so unique and so nutritious has to do with heat. Or rather, the lack of it.

The magic number is 115. When any food item is heated above 115°F, its nutrient density begins to become comprised and degraded. We know this because most vitamins are water soluble, and a significant percentage is lost during cooking. When temperatures are kept low, vitamins and nutrients are preserved. Health enthusiasts and raw foodists also believe the living plant enzymes that aid with digestion are destroyed above 115°F and can no longer aid in the digestive process. Many raw foodists drink a lot of fresh vegetable and green juices, which are packed with nutrients. Released by the juicing process, these nutrients are absorbed extremely quickly, so that your cells can receive a heavy-duty punch of what they need for optimal functioning.

After you've adjusted to eating raw, that's the reason you'll feel the benefits of this lifestyle so quickly. It's also why many raw foodists report weight loss, more energy, improved digestion and health, and an improved, glowing complexion. Their bodies are getting the fuel they need, when they need it—and it shows!

Why a Raw Food Diet Is So Good for Your Body

Eating raw foods or a high-raw diet (80 percent raw and 20 percent cooked foods) allows your digestive system to work efficiently, without stress. When you eat foods that need only minimal energy for your body to break down and absorb, you will have more energy to do whatever it is you want to do—finish a complex project at work, take a dance class, go to the movies with your children, have a date night with your partner—with more vigor. If, on the other hand, you eat processed and nonnutritious fatty or sugar-laden foods, your body goes into digestive overdrive to process and metabolize the food. Your pancreas will churn out large doses of insulin to break down and ab-

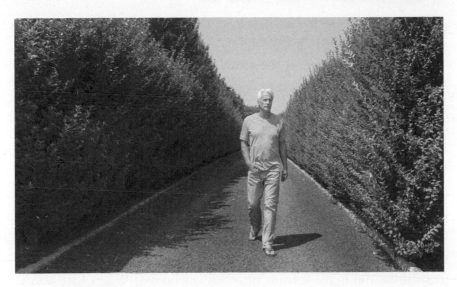

sorb all the sugar, causing spikes in your blood sugar that can leave you feeling tired and cranky and even hungrier, especially when these levels plummet. Worse, any excess sugar not immediately needed by your body will be stored as fat. Who needs that? Not me and not you. Not anyone, in fact!

Let me push this point a little bit more: Let's say you were late for work and barely had time to scarf down a bagel with cream cheese for breakfast. By the time lunch rolls around you're starving, and when your colleagues suggest going to the nearest diner, you happily agree that it's a great idea. You order a cheeseburger and fries for lunch and wolf them down because you're so hungry, and then you can't help ordering a piece of cheesecake for dessert. You go back to the office, but you're suddenly so tired you can barely concentrate and type out the report that's due. So you eat a candy bar for an instant pick-me-up, which works for about twenty minutes, but then all of a sudden you're even more tired and cranky, so you stop for a slice of pizza on the way home to tide you over until dinner.

I know exactly how you'd feel because this is the way I used to eat. I had no idea that eating a hamburger bun made from white flour was basically giving me no viable nutrients, and that the ground beef and gooey melted cheese from the burger would take up to three days to make its way through my intestines.

And I also understand the stress you're under every day and the limited options you might have for eating right. I am an entrepreneur going at a million miles an hour every day, and sometimes—even after eating a high-raw diet for so long—I stop at my local café and have a hummus and guacamole sandwich on sourdough bread. I love it and it tastes great while I'm eating it, but after a while I start to feel irritable and bloated—thanks, primarily, to the highly processed flour in the bread—and always want to crash for a nap. In other words, even the healthiest foods can have adverse reactions for someone like me, who is accustomed to eating raw, not cooked, food. (And hummus is a cooked food unless you make it from sprouted chickpeas!) When I stick to a green smoothie and salad for lunch instead of a sandwich, my energy level skyrockets and my thinking process remains clear.

So let's take a more detailed look at how the digestive process works.

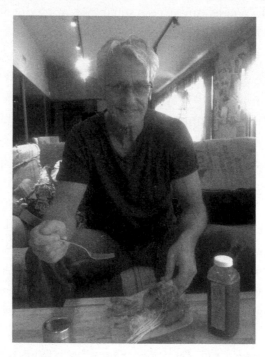

The Good, the Bad, and Your Gut

It's really too bad that most Americans are too squeamish and embarrassed to talk about what's happening in their bellies and guts. Digestion really is a fascinating topic—and an essential one to understand, because once your digestive system stops working properly, you will pay the price for it every day. Digestive problems don't just cause temporary constipation, diarrhea, or terrible bloating and gas. They can cause tremendous discomfort and pain and lead to complicated health issues if you ignore the warning signs that your body is not digesting and eliminating its waste properly.

Digestion is the process by which what you eat and drink is broken down into molecules that can be absorbed into your blood so the nutrients can be carried to the cells throughout your body. Your cells use the nutrients to create energy, and to build and replenish themselves.

Not surprisingly, your body wants the best possible fuel for itself. It wants to work efficiently, too, which is why human beings have evolved to easily store excess calories so they are readily available in times of famine. Unfortunately, in modern society we are rarely famished, so this hyperefficient storage process quickly converts excess calories into fat. If, however, you eat nutrient-dense foods, you will eat less and stay fuller longer because your body will be satiated quickly after you eat and during the digestive process.

Food digestion begins in the mouth—when you chew and the enzymes in your saliva begin their work—and is completed in the small intestine. The leftover liquid waste material is processed through your kidneys and excreted as urine. The solid waste material is solidified in your colon, or large intestine, and then excreted as a bowel movement. How often you need to "go" varies tremendously; what you want is to have consistent elimination so you don't feel plugged up and bloated.

There is a very large difference between how your body metabolizes different foods. Eating a piece of fruit takes, on average, a scant three hours to digest from the time it arrives in your stomach to its further processing in your small intestine. From there to complete elimination can take approximately sixteen to twenty-four hours. Many vegetables take only about six hours.

But red meat can take up to a whopping seventy-two hours to fully digest and eliminate. Yes, that's correct. Up to three days to get that burger out of your body. No wonder you feel so sluggish!

What Are Enzymes and How Do They Impact Your Digestion?

Enzymes are protein molecules that are made by plant and animal cells. There are three categories of enzymes: digestive, metabolic, and food-based. Digestive and metabolic enzymes are produced by your pancreas. Food-based enzymes come from the food you eat.

Enzymes function as catalysts to make the necessary chemical reactions your body needs. What's important for you to understand is that your digestive enzymes help the food you eat to be broken down quickly and effectively in your stomach and small intestine, and then sped off to your bloodstream and cells for nourishment.

Ideally, you should be ingesting the essential food-based enzymes on a daily basis, but if you're eating mostly processed foods that are devoid of any enzymes (or proper nutrients), then you are not getting any of them at all. Worse, the more you eat processed and unhealthy food, especially when it's full of sugar, the more your body needs to overcompensate in order to metabolize it, which further depletes its ability to make more of its own enzymes. And, as you know already, if you cook your food above 115°F, the naturally occurring enzymes in plant and animal cells are destroyed.

Most people don't ever think about enzymes or even know what they do—I certainly didn't! For example, I believed that if I ate a meal with animal protein, such as a steak or a chicken breast, along with some veggies or a salad on the side, the veggies would somehow help me better digest the protein. Don't ask me where that notion came from; suffice to say that I thought it and I believed it and kept on eating whatever I wanted.

But I was very wrong. The raw salad would have contained enough enzymes to digest just that, the salad. It did not contain enough enzymes to digest the animal protein or anything else I would have ingested at that meal. No wonder I felt so awful afterward.

Something else to consider is that your body's own enzyme output decreases as you grow older. This starts for everyone around the age of twenty, and your body's enzyme production continues to decrease by 13 percent every ten years. In addition, as you age, your stomach produces less hydrochloric acid, which is a crucial component in the activation of the digestive enzymes there.

The All-American Sugar Rush

Here's a shocking figure for you: According to the U.S. Department of Agriculture, the average American consumes 156 pounds of sugar per year. No, that is not a typo. Get out your trusty calculator and you'll soon realize that this means that the average adult eater in the United States ingests thirty-one 5-pound bags of sugar in 365 days.

The only person who's happy about this is your dentist!

To understand what sugar does to your body, let me explain the basics of sugar metabolism. Whenever you eat anything, your pancreas releases insulin, the hormone that regulates how you metabolize sugar. Your cells can't process sucrose, which is the ingredient in table sugar, so it must be converted to glucose, which is the sugar that fuels your body.

There are two kinds of carbohydrates. Simple carbohydrates are sugars such as sucrose, high-fructose corn syrup, fructose, dextrose, glucose, honey, malt sugar, and syrup. Though fruit contains fructose, a simple sugar, it is also nutrient-dense and contains fiber, which slows the digestion and absorption of sugar.

Complex carbohydrates include foods such as vegetables, legumes, corn, potatoes, rice, and grain products. Vegetables such as green beans, broccoli, and spinach have less complex carbs but contain a lot of fiber. The best complex carbohydrates to add to your diet are legumes and vegetables, which is why when people say that they're cutting out all carbs, I certainly hope they're not cutting out veggies!

It is a fallacy to think that all simple carbs are bad and all complex carbs are good. A delicious apple is a simple carb and is one of the best foods you can eat. A heaping serving of whole-grain pasta or cereal is a complex carb but is also highly processed and not as good for you as eating a salad or sprouted grain.

The most crucial point to remember is this: Eating raw, living foods in the portions you will read about in part 2 will not cause your blood sugar to spike. You will not have sugar highs or lows, so you will not release extra insulin to compensate for them. Blood sugar levels will remain consistent and stable, allowing you to have maximum energy to fuel your day and maintain a clear and balanced mind.

The reason for this is simple: Whenever you eat a food containing complex carbohydrates as well as fiber and other nutrients, this food is digested slowly and only a minimal amount of insulin is needed to convert the sugar into glucose that will be gradually released into your bloodstream. The key component here is the fiber—it's very difficult to eat a lot of fiber-rich food in one sitting, as your body will rebel! Portion control throughout the day will keep your digestive system working at maximum efficiency.

Eat simple carbohydrates in the form of packaged and processed foods laden with sugar, however, and the opposite happens. Your pancreas goes into emergency mode and pumps out a large amount of insulin to manage all that sugar. I'm sure you know the feeling—it's that sugar rush you get after eating a bagel and coffee with sugar for breakfast, or a handful of cookies as an afternoon snack.

All that insulin and glucose need to go somewhere. As soon as your blood sugar spikes, your insulin levels plummet. You enter into a sugar low or crash, becoming sluggish and cranky, with low energy, often with your mind in a fog and nerves all jittery. You are probably already starting to feel hungry, too, especially for something that is sweet, because your body was primed to digest some real food when all that insulin was released, but it got nothing but empty calories. Yet if you eat more simple carbohydrates, you'll trigger the release of even more insulin, and the whole roller coaster of blood sugar peaks and valleys will start all over again.

When I talk to people who are trying to watch their weight, I explain that the problem with sugar—and one of the biggest contributing factors to the obesity and diabetes epidemics that are sweeping our country—is that it's not just about the few spoonfuls you might put into your coffee in the morning, or what's in the brownie you had for a treat for dessert. Part of the danger comes from food with hidden sugar. If you like those foods and eat them regularly, your taste buds will adjust to the sweetness and you'll find that you crave more and more sweetness without even knowing why.

Sugar is disguised under many different names, such as turbinado sugar, lactose, maltodextrin, maltose, rice syrup, sorbitol, sucrose, fruit juice concentrate, galactose, ethyl maltol, dextrose, dextrin, date sugar, cane sugar; the list could go on. They might sound different—but "pure organic cane sugar" is still plain old white sugar, and the fact that it's organic doesn't make it substantially more nutritious.

One of the worst forms of sugar is high-fructose corn syrup (HFCS), derived from corn. Introduced to the food industry in the 1970s, it is cheap to produce and one of the most prevalent ingredients in all the minimally nutritious sodas, baked goods, cereals, processed foods, and snack foods you want to avoid. Take a good look at the food labels of the packaged items in your pantry and you'll likely be stunned to see HFCS all over the place!

HFCS is not metabolized by your body the same way naturally occurring food sugars are. It takes just one day for your body to fully digest the sugars that are found in fresh fruit and vegetables, but it can take up to four days to digest high-fructose corn syrup. Whenever you eat anything with sugar in it, enzymes in your digestive tract must break down sucrose into a 50/50 ratio of glucose and fructose, which are then absorbed into the body. HFCS contains glucose and fructose in a 45/55 glucose to fructose ratio in an unbound form. Since there is no chemical bond between the glucose and fructose, they are rapidly absorbed into your bloodstream. This triggers an insulin spike, and the whole blood sugar roller coaster I just described starts up again.

If you eat a lot of fat-free products, you're also adding to your sugar load. What happens when you take fat out of a recipe? It has to be replaced with something in order to make it palatable. And what is it usually replaced with? Sugar.

Many of the people I speak to tell me that they've swapped their sugar-laden sodas and foods for those made with artificial sweeteners, but they haven't lost any weight and can't understand why. (Often they are drinking enormous quantities of diet sodas, which are packed with chemicals and should be avoided.) According to the American Diabetes Association, artificial sweeteners such as aspartame, saccharin, and sucralose do not contain carbohydrates and do not have any effect on blood sugar levels. But the problem is that these artificial sweeteners are often paired with other artificial sweeteners that do have an effect—especially those that are sugar alcohols, which are a type of carbohydrate with a chemical structure that partly resembles sugar and partly resembles alcohol. You can identify sugar alcohols on food labels, as they usually end in -ol; look for sorbitol, xylitol, and maltitol. Ingesting sugar alcohols can lead to the same kind of blood sugar spikes I described earlier in this section, creating the same spike-crash cycle and hunger pangs for more sweets.

In addition, eating or drinking foods with fake sugars often doesn't give you the same satisfaction as the real thing. You don't get the same "mouth feel" and you don't get the same satiety factor, and so you may end up craving the sugary food you wanted to eat in the first place with even more urgency.

My advice is to stay away from any artificial sweeteners in anything you eat or drink. You will find many great natural sweetener options in chapter 7, including coconut nectar, maple syrup, honey, agave, and green leaf stevia.

PROTEIN SOURCES

How Much Protein Does Your Body Really Need?

The number one question I am asked is whether it is possible to get enough protein on a raw diet. It's also the biggest argument that proponents on either side of the raw debate have about making the switch from the standard American diet to a raw, vegan diet.

Protein is important for maintaining muscle and bone mass, for keeping the immune system strong, and for preventing fatigue. A protein contains amino acids (there are twenty-two) and can either be complete or incomplete. A complete protein source contains all nine of the twenty-two essential amino acids your body can't produce on its own; an incomplete protein source may not contain all the essential amino acids, or have too little of one, which limits the ability of the food to make its other amino acids available to you. This is why many cultures combine foods with incomplete proteins, giving your body all the amino acids it needs in the proper form. The best example of this is rice and beans.

Here's where the protein situation gets interesting. The daily recommended allowance of protein ranges from 41 to 61 grams, depending on your body mass and the amount of physical activity you do in a day. If you look on a food label, it will state that for an average person eating two thousand calories per day, the daily recommended allowance of protein is 50 grams. Bear in mind, however, that protein needs vary. If you are an endurance runner your protein intake should be much higher than that of a sedentary person, and if you are pregnant or nursing your protein needs will also increase.

Before you go raw keep a food diary for a day, eating foods such as canned tuna, beans, or dairy that have a detailed food nutrition label on them. Then tally up the total grams of protein. If your protein consumption is above average, you are not alone!

It's been estimated that in America the average eater consumes 50 percent more protein than the daily recommended amount. Two cups of milk, for example, contain 16 grams of protein; a small tin of sardines contains nearly 20 grams; and one cup of canned beans contains 18 grams. If you consume them in one meal, you likely will have met your protein requirement for the day. But what about the other two meals, or snacks? What happens to all that extra protein? Your body isn't capable of storing protein the way it stores fat, so the excess is excreted through your kidneys. If you eat a lot of steak, this can give you some very expensive urine!

Take a look at the vegan protein sources listed here. I was surprised when I started reading about raw foods to see how many plant-based sources of protein there are. So rest assured that when you are eating a balanced plant-based diet, your protein needs will be fulfilled.

THE BEST VEGETARIAN AND VEGAN PROTEIN SOURCES

Nuts and seeds:	almonds, cashews, chia seeds, hemp seeds, pecans, pistachios, sunflower seeds, pumpkin seeds, walnuts
Grains:	brown rice, oatmeal, quinoa, seitan, wheat germ
Legumes:	beans, lentils, peanuts, peas, soybeans
Vegetables:	avocados, broccoli, carrots, kale and other dark leafy greens, mushrooms, romaine lettuce, tomatoes
Fruit:	apples, bananas, oranges, strawberries
Seaweed:	spirulina

Now that you know how easy it is to obtain your necessary amount of protein from plant-based sources, let's take a look at how dairy and animal protein affect your body.

Got Milk? Are You Sure?

I was raised in a culture where milk and dairy products were considered an essential part of every child's diet. Even now, milk is always served as a part of daily school lunches. I loved cheese and ice cream and never thought I could stop eating dairy, so one of the biggest shocks I had when I went raw is how many satisfying alternatives to dairy there are and how little I missed it.

One of the biggest issues with dairy products in our world today has to do with the mass consumption of milk products and how milk is produced.

Dairy cows can produce only a certain amount of milk each day, so to meet our country's growing demand for milk and milk products, most farmers give their cows bovine growth hormone (BGH) to make them mature faster and produce more milk. There is grave concern from groups such as the Consumers Union and the Cancer Prevention Coalition that this practice is harmful to humans. Here's why: Cows given this hormone are more prone to udder infections and reproductive problems. How are they treated? With antibiotics. Where do the antibiotics go? Into the milk the cows are producing as well as into our ecosystem when they're excreted. Who drinks the milk or eats the cheese or drinks the water? You do.

Overuse of bovine antibiotics has devastating implications for your health and for global health. Over time, bacteria that cause illness can develop a resistance to these antibiotics. We're seeing this already with tuberculosis and some sexually transmitted diseases. We're also seeing this in hospitals with the rise of superbugs that are lethal to patients who are already seriously ill and can't fight off infections. (Needless to say, you should never, ever take antibiotics unless you truly need them, and if and when they are prescribed, you must follow the directions on the pill bottle and always take all of the medication; taking less kills only the weakest bacteria. You never need antibiotics if you have a virus, such as the common cold or the flu, since antibiotics are effective only against bacterial infections, and viruses are not bacteria!)

Another serious concern with injecting BGH into cows is that it may cause them to produce more of another hormone called insulin-like growth factor–1, or IGF-1. Animal studies have shown that elevation of this hormone could increase the risk for certain cancers in humans, particularly breast and colon cancer. If you are going to incorporate milk into your diet from time to time, make sure you read the label carefully and purchase only milk that clearly states it is BGH-free.

Something else to think about is that dairy might not be such a good food for your body, even though it contains calcium and protein and other trace nutrients. (Bear in mind, too, that unless they are fat-free or reduced fat, milk and cheese contain a lot of fat, along with little fiber, which is why you can unwittingly eat a lot of cheese without it filling you up.) Many people have a degree of lactose intolerance without even realizing it. For them, eating or drinking dairy products can cause unpleasant and uncomfortable gastrointestinal symptoms, such as bloating, cramping, gas, and diarrhea, ranging in severity. Estimates on how many people are lactose intolerant vary greatly. Among Asians, Africans, Latinos, and Native Americans, who until recently rarely ate dairy products and therefore have less genetic adaptability to it, the figure is very high—up to 90 percent! (Lactose intolerance is different from an allergic reaction to dairy products, which can be life threatening.) Casein, the most abundant protein in cow's milk, is also used to make adhesives such as glue. If casein can help make objects stick together, think about what it is doing to your body!

If you are experiencing bloating, cramping, gas, or diarrhea, an easy way to test your intolerance levels is with an elimination diet. Stop eating all dairy for seven days. Then, introduce one kind of product, such as milk or cheese, at a time. If you are lactose intolerant you should notice symptoms within thirty minutes to two hours.

Now that you know what dairy does to your body, you start rethinking (as I did) how much of it you regularly ingest, and how prudent it might be to start looking for equally delicious and satisfying alternatives.

THE CALCIUM CONUNDRUM

One of the biggest worries people have is getting enough calcium if they stop eating dairy products.

It is also one of the most easily alleviated once you realize how

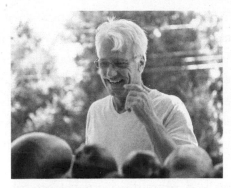 many alternative sources of calcium there are. Oftentimes, the calcium from these alternative sources is more readily absorbed by your body than calcium from dairy. Dark green leafy vegetables such as broccoli, kale, and collard greens have absorption rates of more than 50 percent, compared with about 32 percent for milk. These veggies also contain beneficial phytochemicals and antioxidants that dairy products do not.

In addition, according to a 2005 study, "Calcium, Dairy Products, and Bone Health in Children and Young Adults: A Reevaluation of the Evidence," dairy products can also increase the risk of urinary excretion of calcium; this is due to the sodium, sulfur-containing amino acid, and phosphorus content of dairy products.

In short: Eat your dark leafy greens, and if you're still worried or have a family history of osteoporosis or other bone issues, be sure to discuss your concerns with your physician to see if a supplement might be warranted. Don't use calcium as an excuse to scarf down lots of sugar-laden ice cream!

The Meat of the Matter

William Castelli, M.D., was one of the directors of the Framingham Heart Study, the longest-running clinical study in medical history. It has been tracking health information about the heart disease of adult participants since 1948. The researchers meticulously document the data about each participant's lifestyle, especially their dietary and exercise habits. Dr. Castelli was famously quoted about the heart disease epidemic in this country: "If Americans adopted a vegetarian diet, the whole thing would disappear."

There is plenty of research to support Dr. Castelli's theory. In

February 2005, for example, a major study published in the *American Journal of Epidemiology* confirmed the link between animal products and heart disease, concluding that among twenty-nine thousand participants, those who ate the most meat were also at the greatest risk of heart disease. Dr. Linda E. Kelemen, the scientist who led the study, concluded that not all proteins are created equal. Her colleagues found that a high intake of protein from non-animal sources—such as nuts and beans—lowers the risk of heart disease by 30 percent.

The connection between meat and heart disease is cholesterol, a waxy substance found in fats and in all the cells of your body. It is transported in your bloodstream. Everyone has it in varying levels, as cholesterol is necessary for your body to function.

The two kinds of cholesterol that are typically measured during a routine exam are LDL (low-density lipoprotein) and HDL (high-density lipoprotein). HDL cholesterol is considered "good" cholesterol, as it transports fat lipids to your liver (and away from your heart) to be reprocessed, which helps keep arteries free from buildup. LDL is considered the "bad" kind, since it can form fibrous, fatty deposits called plaque. When too much plaque builds up inside the walls of your arteries in a condition known as atherosclerosis, the arteries get clogged. Blood flow to the heart can be greatly diminished, which leads to heart disease and heart attacks.

According to the National Cholesterol Education Program, borderline high cholesterol is a total cholesterol level of 200–239. Anything that registers as 240 and above is considered very high. When looking at LDL levels only, borderline high LDL levels are 130–159; high levels are 160–189; and 190 and above is considered very high. The average meat eater's cholesterol level is a dangerous 210—while the average vegetarian's cholesterol level is 161, and the average vegan's cholesterol level is 133.

What causes excess cholesterol to be formed? There are many factors, including heredity (which you can't control), inactivity (which you can control), and your diet (which you can also control), particularly if you consume a lot of food and drinks containing saturated fat.

Saturated fats are fatty acids that are solid at room temperature, such as Crisco, lard, or the marbled white streaks and chunks you see in a raw steak. Red meat is one of the top sources of saturated fat, which is why one of the world's most respected nutrition experts, Dr. Caldwell Esselstyn, Jr., who has been associated with the Cleveland Clinic since 1968, has found that when people switch from a meat-heavy diet to a vegetarian diet, heart disease can be reversed as well as prevented in the first place.

I learned from Dr. Esselstyn's studies and my own research that eating a plant-based diet will, for many people, reduce cholesterol levels. When I was eating my old crummy diet, where I thought nothing of scarfing down cheesesteaks, burritos, and rib-eye steaks (can you tell I liked my meat?), washed down by several glasses of vintage red wine at business dinners several times a week, my cholesterol skyrocketed. My physician looked at the alarming numbers, gave me a lecture, and told me that I needed to take a statin drug, which can be effective at lowering cholesterol but also can have potent side effects. Talk about a wake-up call. I wasn't about to take medication when the solution was so much healthier and better for me.

After only three months on a raw food diet, I went back to my doctor for blood work. He was stunned (and thrilled) that my numbers had come back to normal and my cholesterol was at a very healthy level. In fact, my total cholesterol had dropped by a whopping forty points in three months. That was the power of raw in action.

Cutting meat out of your diet entirely is only for hard-core raw foodists. As you know already, sometimes I get a serious craving for a steak, and when that happens I eat it and I certainly do enjoy it. Being able to eat and enjoy small amounts of meat is an integral part of my 80/20 plan, which you'll read about in part 2 of this book. Whenever you feel like eating meat, try to do your utmost to eat only high-quality hormone-free organic meat. After a meat day, I always ensure that my intake of fresh green juices and smoothies is high to help replenish my body with healthy nutrients and minerals.

ACID VERSUS ALKALINE

Something you'll hear discussed often in the raw food community is acid versus alkaline. Every human body has a normal pH (derived from power plus hydrogen) level in their blood, which is the balance between acid and alkaline. Paying attention to your body's pH is important in maintaining a healthy diet, as it's best for you to have a pH of about 7.4, which is slightly more on the alkaline side. A pH level of less than 7 indicates a higher acid level.

It is very easy to test your body's pH level with test strips you can purchase at most health food stores. You can also get free test strips from my website; I will mail them directly to you at no charge. The test can be done with saliva or urine, and results will appear within fifteen seconds. As always, follow package directions when testing for pH so the results will be accurate.

A diet that is high in acidity will decrease your body's ability to absorb minerals and other nutrients, decrease the energy production in your cells, and decrease your ability to repair damaged cells. If your body is very acidic, it will not be able to take in and use available oxygen to stay healthy. If, on the other hand, it's more alkaline, oxygen will be delivered to the cells as needed. Because most people don't eat enough high-alkaline fresh fruits and vegetables, their bodies become too acidic. This adds an additional layer of stress, as the body will always strive to maintain a normal pH level.

If your body is too acidic, you might have some or many of the following symptoms: low energy, chronic fatigue, excess mucus production, nasal congestion, frequent colds and infections, nervousness, stress, irritability, anxiety, headaches, muscle pain or joint pain, arthritis, weight gain, and kidney stones. I had a lot of these symptoms until I went raw and got my own pH levels back on track.

To bring your pH level back to a more normal range you should concentrate on eating a diet that is 80 percent alkaline-forming foods. Once you are back to normal, you should eat a diet of 65–75 percent alkaline-forming foods.

HIGH ALKALINE OR ALKALINE-FORMING FOODS

Fruit: blackberries, cantaloupe, honeydew melon, limes, nectarines,
      papaya, pineapple, raspberries, strawberries, tangerines,
      watermelon

Vegetables: asparagus, broccoli, celery, collard greens, endive, garlic,
      kale, mustard greens, onions, parsnips, spinach, sweet potato,
      winter squash, yams

Nuts, seeds, and spices: chestnuts, ginger root, pumpkin seeds, parsley,
      sea salt

Vinegars: umeboshi vinegar

UNDERSTANDING THE DIFFERENCES BETWEEN RAW, COOKED, AND PROCESSED FOODS

Raw foods are just that: uncooked and, if heated, not heated above 115°F. Some experts will argue that no nutrients at all are lost during cooking or flash freezing—and I obviously disagree, as do those in the raw food community. I think it's safe to say that cooking will have some effect on nutrient levels, and it is certain that your body's ability to absorb the nutrients decreases dramatically when food is cooked.

Bear in mind that not only are raw foods laden with vitamins, minerals, and micronutrients, but they also add oxygen and chlorophyll to your diet. Green vegetables are primarily composed of water, which is mostly oxygen by weight. When cooked at high temperatures, they lose the chlorophyll and the water is evaporated. You see this process in action if you sauté or roast veggies, which shrink down dramatically in size the longer they are heated. You also see it when you cook green veggies and their bright color turns gray. It is believed that chlorophyll is lost after about twenty minutes of cooking, which is why I recommend that you either steam green veggies for less than five minutes or eat them raw.

Chlorophyll is the pigment that gives plants their green color and is found in most plants and algae; it facilitates photosynthesis, the process by which plants use sunlight to synthesize food (energy) from carbon dioxide and water. It is rich in minerals as well as amino acids, which are the building blocks of protein. Even better, because chlorophyll's pH levels are exactly the same as those found in our blood, eating foods high in chlorophyll help your body stabilize its alkalinity. There are other benefits as well: Chlorophyll acts as a natural detoxifier in the body. It helps the blood deliver oxygen to the cells of the body and neutralizes free radicals (see below) that cause cell damage. It is also a natural deodorizer and can help neutralize bad breath or body odors (which is why you'll find it in many mouthwashes and deodorants).

What Happens to Food When You Heat It?

Heating your food to very high temperatures, which happens when you roast, grill, or deep-fry, not only destroys nearly all enzymes, vitamins, and minerals but has potentially even more harmful effects.

Cooking any animal protein at high temperatures creates carcinogens called heterocyclic amines. Studies at the National Cancer Institute have shown that they can greatly increase cancer risk in humans, as they damage DNA only after they are metabolized by specific enzymes in the body. Fried meat has been linked to an increased risk of hormone-related cancers in women and an even higher risk of prostate cancer for men. Not only that, but grilling chars and burns meat, especially the fat; this process produces a high level of a carcinogenic substance called nitrosamine, which has been linked to colon cancer.

In addition, cooking food changes some of the active compounds found within them, most notably antioxidants. "Antioxidants" and "free radicals" are words that are often used when talking about food or skin care, but most people don't quite understand what they mean.

Free radicals are damaged cells that can become problematic. From a scientist's perspective, free radicals are defined as atoms or groups of atoms containing an unpaired number of electrons, formed when oxygen interacts with certain molecules. Because they are missing a critical molecule, they are highly reactive while in desperate pursuit of another molecule with which they can bond, and they are particularly damaging when they interact with cellular components such as DNA or cell membranes. If they finally latch on to a molecule within a cell itself, the cell can be injured and its DNA altered, setting off a chain reaction of abnormal cell growth and reproduction.

Antioxidants are molecules that can safely interact with free radicals and stop this damaging, disease-causing chain reaction. The principal micronutrient antioxidants are vitamin E, beta-carotene, and vitamin C; they must be consumed via the food you eat, as your body can't manufacture them.

Does all of this mean you can never enjoy a grilled steak or burger without worrying again? Of course not (unless you eat blackened catfish every day of your life!). It just means you need to be aware of what cooking can do, and how it might affect your health over the span of your lifetime.

Time to Zap the Zapper

One last thought—you might want to look at your microwave with a jaundiced eye if not get rid of it altogether. I don't think anyone has ever done the math in a double-blind study, but it may well be true that the onset of our current obesity epidemic started around the time that microwave use became commonplace in the American kitchen. Why? Because it made "cooking" so much easier and faster—and the convenient packaged foods we love to pull out of the freezer and microwave are often packed with sugar, salt, and saturated fat. It's something to think about. Besides, do you know what happens when you microwave food? Microwave ovens heat food through creating molecular friction. This might zap your food or your cold cup of coffee quickly, which is great when you're in a hurry, but by doing so it destroys the delicate molecules of vitamins and phytonutrients that are naturally found in foods—and especially in plant-based foods.

Microwaving also causes a problem if you heat food in the packaging it came in, or in another plastic container. The unusual heating process of the microwave leeches numerous toxic chemicals out of Styrofoam and plastic, releasing dioxins and other toxins that are known carcinogens into your food. One of the biggest offenders is bisphenol A, or BPA, which is an estrogen-like compound found in many plastics. It was declared a toxic substance in Canada in 2010, and only in 2012 was it finally banned from use in the manufacturing of plastic baby bottles in the United States. That is scant comfort to the generations of parents who trusted that the bottles they were using for their precious infants were safe. When it comes to chemicals and packaging, it's often hard to know what to believe.

When I read up on this, I immediately got rid of my microwave. I no longer believe that the convenience of instant heating is worth the downside of potentially wreaking havoc on your health.

How Dehydration Makes Eating Raw So Much More Flavorful

Most raw foodists "cook" their food in dehydrators, which keeps enzymes and nutrients intact.

Food dehydrators remove the moisture from food and help it remain edible longer. As you begin to read more about dehydration, you will see varying temperatures as the limit for dehydration. I have seen them as low as 106°F and as high as 118°F. I dehydrate nearly everything at 115°F degrees and feel that is an appropriate temperature for preserving vitamins, minerals, and enzymes.

Dehydration is a fantastic technique when you eat raw, as it will give you that crunch that you might miss as you first venture into the raw food world. Some of the best things to make are crackers, breads, pizza crusts, raw popcorn, veggies, granola, and chips. You will find a few recipes in this book to experiment with, but of course you don't need to invest in a dehydrator in order to eat a satisfyingly crunchy and scrumptious raw diet.

I hope you are intrigued and excited to read more about the benefits of eating raw, and then begin to follow my 8-week plan in part 2. Every time temptation sneaks in as you move throughout the next 8 weeks, come back to this chapter and remind yourself about what your old diet did to your body! But first, take a look at the next chapter, where I'll show you precisely how and why a healthy raw diet will make you feel and look so much better.

2

THE BRILLIANT BENEFITS OF PLANT-BASED EATING

Now that you know why raw food is so good for you, let's take a look at how eating a predominantly raw diet will make you feel.

BETTER HEALTH AND VITALITY: A DIET HIGH IN FRESH, RAW NUTRIENTS MAKES YOU FEEL GREAT

Hippocrates lived in ancient Greece and is considered the father of medicine. When doctors graduate from medical school, they take a modernized version of the Hippocratic oath. The part that resonates most strongly with me is "I will prevent disease whenever I can, for prevention is preferable to cure."

He also said, "Let food be thy medicine, let medicine be thy food." Now that was one smart guy!

But you know as well as I do that our modern diet has changed radically from what Hippocrates's patients, or even our great-grandparents, ate. Before modern refrigerators, freezers, mass manufacturers, plastic packaging, and microwave ovens came along, consumers went to local markets and purchased fresh food. The only kind of packaged food available came in metal cans or glass bottles; it was much more expensive than fresh food and usually considered a treat.

Fast-forward to now. Processed, not fresh, food dominates so much of the average diet. Sure, it's awfully easy to open a box and whip up a quick meal, but you might not be aware of how much is sacrificed for speed and convenience.

Some processed food, such as frozen vegetables—which have been flash frozen shortly after being harvested and cleaned—is nearly as nutritious as fresh. (How you cook it, however, will affect the nutrient levels; steaming it at low temperatures is best.) In general, however, raw food that has not been processed retains a much higher level of nutrients and antioxidants. Put all other food through typical processing—by which I mean removing much of the fiber and essential vitamins and minerals—and the food is much less nutritious. You don't just have to worry about what's been added to it, but also what's been taken away. Antioxidants, fiber, and good fats are an essential part of a healthy diet, but most processed foods are missing these good ingredients.

Take the familiar potato. The peel is a good source of vitamin C, vitamin B_6, copper, potassium, and zinc, and the flesh is a great source of fiber. But when the potato is turned into potato chips, the peel is stripped away, the flesh is fried in unhealthy oil, and salt and synthetic seasonings and chemical preservatives are sometimes added to the bag for "freshness." The result is a chip that contains a lot of crunch and not much else. That's why a normal eater can eat one fiber-rich potato at dinner and feel full, but you can easily consume an entire bag of potato chips before you've realized it—and still be hungry.

So many other foods that are processed have little to no nutrient density. Converting brown rice into white rice strips off the kernel and hull that contain most of its fiber, selenium, and magnesium. Making oatmeal "instant" and adding lots of sugar to the packets makes it a simple carbohydrate, whereas a batch of steel-cut oats dehydrated into granola will give your body a huge dollop of fiber and keep you filled for hours.

Take a look at some of the ingredients listed on a typical box of macaroni and cheese: "enriched macaroni product," cheese sauce mix with whey, modified food starch, milk fat, salt, milk protein concentrate, cheese, medium chain triglycerides, silicon dioxide as an anti-caking agent, enzyme modified butter oil, yellow 5, yellow 6, yeast, and much more. Now, compare that with macaroni and cheese you could make yourself with whole grain pasta, good cheese, and fresh milk. Both take the exact same amount of time to cook. But which one is so much better for your kids? Better yet—try Brad's Raw Mac and Cheese (page 173).

Worse, many processed foods are full of hidden sugars, chemicals, and fats that are added solely to improve "taste." As you know, eating too much fatty food is a contributing factor to heart disease and other cardiovascular problems. Eating too much of any food that is not good for you leads to obesity, which is at epidemic levels in this country.

In addition, processed food often contains harmful trans fats. This kind of fat increases your levels of bad cholesterol (LDL) and decreases your levels of good cholesterol (HDL).

These foods also contain very high levels of sodium. Your body needs sodium, of course, to regulate your blood pressure and maintain your body's fluid balance—you'd die without it. Many of the raw foods you'll be eating contain sodium naturally, such as celery (which is a great base for fresh juice). But most Americans are so used to eating salty food that they overdo it on a daily basis. It drives me crazy when I see people adding salt to food before they've even tasted it, and it makes me even more crazy when I know how overloaded processed foods are with totally unnecessarily high levels of sodium.

Last but not least, many processed foods contain high-fructose corn syrup. You already read about how bad this stuff is in chapter 1. It raises the risk of heart disease, diabetes, and obesity. You'll soon see how reducing your consumption of sugar, especially in the form of high-fructose corn syrup—and eliminating it completely during the plan—will make you feel so much better.

Eating a raw food diet might not guarantee that you'll never experience another cold or bout of the flu again, but by eating nutrient-dense raw food, your body will be strong and healthy and better equipped to fight off a potential infection.

I used to get colds and coughs all the time, especially because I was always traveling and breathing in the dry, dirty air of planes and hotels and not taking care of myself. I rarely get sick now, and when I do it's only for a day or so. If I'm starting to feel low or like a cold is coming on, I normally up my intake of vitamin C through fresh juices for a few days. If I can, I take a few "hot" yoga classes to help speed up the detoxification process by sweating.

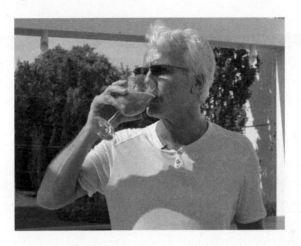

BETTER DIGESTION: ENZYME-RICH RAW FOODS MAKE DIGESTION LESS OF A STRAIN ON YOUR SYSTEM

Ever notice how you want to take a nap after a large meal, even if you weren't particularly sleepy beforehand? It's because your body literally can't process all those calories and do whatever else it is you want to do at the same time. In other words, if your body needs to expend a lot of energy on digesting the stuff you ate or drank, of course you are going to feel tired and want to conk out!

Did you know that 46 percent of Americans suffer from poor digestion issues? That's nearly half the population. And do you know why? Because the processed foods they're eating on a daily basis are overtaxing their digestive systems. I'm talking about excessive burping, chronic bloating, diarrhea, gas, constipation, heartburn, and acid reflux. These are all very unsubtle signs that your poor stomach and intestines are trying to talk to you. If they could put it into words, they'd say, "Please, I'm begging you, can you just feed us a nice green salad and a tall, cool, luscious green smoothie? Really, we'll feel so much better."

A perfect example of someone who struggled for years with poor digestion is Jaime, who works with me.

JAIME'S STORY

Ever since I was a child I can remember having terrible problems with my stomach and digestive system. I'd be constipated for days on end, with awful pain and bloating. By the time I got to high school I'd already seen multiple gastroenterologists and other specialists, and they couldn't figure out what was wrong with me. One doctor prescribed a muscle relaxer; your stomach, as you know, is a muscle. I'd slide a little pill under my tongue, and within twenty minutes the stabbing pains in my stomach would ease—only because the pill attacked the symptoms, not the cause.

All the tests I took kept coming back negative. So my doctors told me to keep on taking the little pills whenever I needed to. I was popping them like candy. In fact, I panicked if I ever left the house without that pill bottle in my purse!

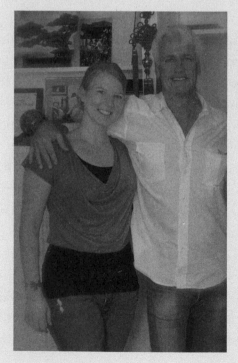

Not one of the medical professionals I'd been seeing for years ever asked me what I ate, or remotely considered that my pain and stomach problems could be related to my diet.

My stomach problems didn't prevent me from getting a business degree in college. When the company I was working for was sold and I was laid off—along with 90 percent of my colleagues—I realized it was a blessing in disguise, enabling me to take some time to figure out my next career move. I decided to go to New York and train as a yoga teacher; I wanted to immerse myself in the holistic lifestyle I was starting to learn about and loved. I signed up for a program at the Institute for Integrative Nutrition, thinking that it would give me additional training about healthy eating—and help me figure out what was wrong with my stomach. Each week we were taught a new dietary theory, and I would experiment with my food intake to see how my body felt.

Not long after that, Brad hired me to do sales and marketing. He asked me to do a juice fast with him, and suggested I go totally raw for a few weeks first to start cleansing my body.

Brad was incredibly encouraging. We'd go into the kitchen at the end of the night after they were done dehydrating the kale, and we'd make enormous salads to pack with us for our road trips to sell the kale chips. I totally fell in love with Brad's famous red bell pepper dressing.

Once the juice fast part of the cleanse started I was tired, weak, and sometimes a little cranky, but that lasted only for three days. To tell you the truth, it really didn't bother me so much because at the same time I realized that my stomach had stopped hurting. I'd been so accustomed to living with chronic digestive problems that it took me a while to real-ize my pipes were working normally. I'd actually completely given up on ever feeling good and pain-free again.

After I finished the raw foods cleanse, it was a no-brainer to stick to a high-raw diet. When I eat cooked food, it's often something like qui-noa, a portobello mushroom burger, or my own type of veggie burger. It's really the essence of the program in this book—to add to your diet, not subtract from it. If you want to have a beautiful salad and cook a steak, then eat it and enjoy it. I know how much raw helped my body, because I've never had those stomach pains again. I really was shocked that something as simple as proper nutrition could rid me of a problem I thought I'd be stuck with for life. Shocked—and thrilled!

If you would like to connect with Jaime and ask her questions about her experiences, you can find her through the Nourished Community, our online community support forum, along with the stories and blogs of others who overcame health issues by changing their lifestyle and diet. Visit bradsrawfoods.com to connect.

And like Jaime, during the Simply Raw part of the plan, you'll get all the healthy calories, nutrients, and enzymes your body needs. Your digestion will improve and your energy will increase when your diet is balanced with cultured, fermented foods such as kimchi, pickles, and kombucha, which add probiotics—the healthy bacteria found in your gut that are necessary for the efficient functioning of your intestines.

Drinking fresh juices each day will also give your energy a boost and your digestive system a break. They're a great way to start your day because they allow your digestive system to stay in rest mode and work on elimination prior to ingesting your first meal. Think about it this way: To make juice you need to use a decent amount of produce. I don't know anyone who can get up and happily eat four stalks of celery, three large handfuls of spinach, a handful of parsley, and an apple before 9 a.m. I know I couldn't. It's much easier to juice all of those ingredients and give your body that shot of health, greens, and nutrients when you start your morning. Not that you don't need fiber, of course—which is why I advocate that you eat a mixture of fresh juice, smoothies, salads, and healthy meals throughout your day.

MY FRIEND EVA NORMAN'S STORY

I used to have digestive problems, with a lot of pain and cramping. At times I felt so bad that I was afraid I would not be able to work a full-time job.

The doctors I consulted wanted me to take medication that has severe side effects, and I didn't want to do that. So I started doing a lot of reading about nutrition, and started an elimination diet. I found that eating dairy products made me feel one hundred times worse. I tried following an extremely strict diet, with no dairy, meat, sugar, or salt; sometimes it helped, and it made me even more convinced that how I was eating was the trigger for my gut pain. Once I was able to go 100 percent raw, 100 percent of my symptoms disappeared. I was finally able to drop the idea that I had anything wrong with me. It was just the food!

Then, during a highly stressful period in my life, I ate some raw food and some cooked food. I wasn't having my terrible old symptoms, but I realized that if I don't watch what I eat, they start creeping back in, and I also gained weight, which nobody ever likes! I've accepted the fact that I need to pack it in and pack it out—I bring my food with me. I'm getting better with understanding how much food I need.

I don't find the food prep to be time consuming because in the raw food world you can do it at different levels. It's fun to do the complicated recipes, but I prefer the simpler foods when I'm busy. I start cutting up food to prepare some fabulous thing, and then if I don't have time I just eat it as is!

BETTER WEIGHT LOSS: YOU WON'T GO HUNGRY AGAIN

There are many reasons why raw foods help the pounds disappear.

Fiber Is Filling

Many fruits and nearly all vegetables are naturally low in calories and contain high amounts of fiber, which is what makes you feel full. High-fiber foods provide volume and take longer for your body to digest, so it won't be sending out signals to your brain that it needs more food.

You'll find many tips throughout about which raw foods are the most filling. For example, chia seeds are a superfood that will help you feel full, and they have the added benefit of being an amazing cleanser for your digestive tract. Hemp seeds are another superfood that you can easily add to your smoothies, and they are especially easy to digest. Other examples of high-fiber foods that help you feel full are broccoli, carrots, Brussels sprouts, raspberries, bananas, and oranges.

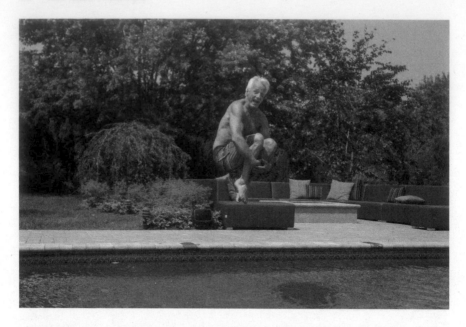

Cravings for Junk Will Go Away

Sometimes you reach for things unwittingly because they make you feel satiated and full right away (even though that feeling of fullness quickly wears off). I know it's hard to believe if you've been addicted to certain kinds of foods or snacks most of your life—I used to gobble down carbohydrates such as bagels, muffins, breads, and pastas without thinking—but you honestly will not miss them. After a while, I completely lost my taste for sugar. Believe me, I am the last person who ever would have said that only a few years ago!

Even better, the more you eat nutrient-dense foods, the more your body will crave what it knows is good for it, and the cravings you used to have for crummy food will diminish. Right now, your body is lacking nutrients and is trying to get them any which way it can. When you start my meal plan by adding a simple green smoothie first thing in the morning, you'll give your body the nutrition it's been needing, and you'll be set up for eating success for the rest of the day.

Eating Good Fats Won't Make You Fat!

Why did fat become the enemy? Your body can't function properly without fats. Without fats your skin will look lifeless, your muscles will hang limp, you'll have no energy, and your brainpower will diminish tremendously. And while good fats, such as coconut oil, are high in calories, they are incredibly filling. You literally can't eat a lot of good fat because your stomach will balk!

You'll Be Getting Rid of Toxins

Toxins are poisonous substances produced within living cells or organisms; they're found in our homes, at work, in the air we breathe, in the soil, and, of course, in the over-processed food we eat. They can kill you quickly (if you get bitten by a snake or if you breathe in contaminated air), or they can affect how your body functions, slowly, over time (if you eat and drink a lot of food containing ingredients that aren't good for you). Even healthy substances, such as fat-soluble vitamins, can be toxic if consumed in enormous quantities.

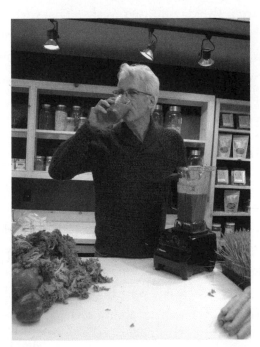

Over time, toxins from our foods and environment are stored in our bodies. This is because most environmental toxins are fat soluble, which means they are stored in your fat cells. This creates a double whammy of stressing your thyroid (which regulates your metabolism) while affecting your appetite (often increasing it). A slower metabolism means you need and burn fewer calories, and you can gain weight even when eating the same amount of food you usually do. A normal or high-functioning metabolism, on the other hand, helps you lose weight.

In a 2008 study published in the journal *Acta Paediatrica*, researchers from Barcelona's Municipal Institute of Medical Research found that babies born with higher levels of pesticide were twice as likely to be obese by age six. Another study published in the *International Journal of Obesity* in 2010 concluded that participants who reported a large amount of weight loss had about 50 percent higher levels of six organic pollutants in their blood serum than participants who had large weight gains. In other words, these two studies demonstrated that toxins can be released from fat tissue during short-term weight loss.

When you start to eat 100 percent raw, you may feel like you have the flu, or you might have headaches and fatigue. These symptoms can last anywhere from five days to two weeks. That's why your first step will be the first phase, Prepare—a two-week time where you gently transition to raw. Even if you're still feeling a bit crummy, please understand that when you start to feel this way, you are actually doing something amazing for your body.

High-Alkaline Food Helps You Lose Weight

A healthy body has a pH balance of around 7.4, which is slightly alkaline. Most people, however, eat too many foods that tend toward acidity, including animal proteins such as bacon, beef, and milk, as well as poor quality sweeteners such as high-fructose corn syrup and white table sugar. Alcohol is also very acidic, as are aspirin, tobacco, and coffee. Too much acidity decreases your body's ability to absorb minerals and other nutrients, decreases its ability to repair damaged cells, decreases its energy production ability within the cells themselves, and decreases its ability to detoxify heavy metals such as mercury and lead, if you have been exposed to them.

A high-acid diet triggers your body to bind the acidity in your fat cells and store it under the skin, often in your stomach, thighs, arms, and under your chin. Your body is smart enough to know that this acid needs to be kept away from your vital organs. Doesn't sound so nice, does it?

If, on the other hand, you start to remove high-acid foods from your diet and switch to a balanced diet that is higher in alkaline foods, it will prevent all this acidity from being stored in your fat cells. Our bodies naturally keep large alkaline reserves to balance a diet containing acid-producing foods. When these reserves are depleted beyond a certain ratio, it creates an environment that allows yeast, viruses, and parasites to thrive, which can contribute to conditions such as chronic fatigue, allergies, arthritis, and more. If the body becomes too acidic, it will start using its reserves of sodium, magnesium, potassium, and calcium, which can create serious mineral deficiencies. Finding this balance is important for overall health, and will help you to lose weight.

It is recommended that your diet consists of an 80/20 ratio of alkaline foods to acidic foods. You can easily gauge your alkalinity by testing yourself each day. A pH level under 7.4 means you do not have enough alkaline reserves in your body. If so, eat more alkaline foods as you continue your daily pH testing, including green leafy vegetables, avocados, almond milk, young coconut water, wheatgrass, green smoothies, seaweeds, and pineapple.

Bear in mind, though, that when you first start the plan, you might test higher in acidity, especially if you are changing your diet for the first time. If you test your pH every day, by week 3, which is the start of the 100 percent raw portion of the diet, you will start to notice your pH rising every day. By sticking to the plan you will be able to naturally alkalinize your body, and I hope that will keep you motivated to stay on the raw food track.

ARTHUR'S STORY

Twelve years ago I was a successful Wall Street guy. I had four beautiful children under the age of eight and had gone through a long, difficult divorce. I worked hard, I took care of my kids, and I took good care of myself and exercised, but emotionally I was a mess and the toxicity of the stress I was under started taking a tremendous toll on my immune system.

One day, after a run in Central Park, I spiked a very high fever. I thought it was the flu, but when my fever didn't go down after a few days I went to the doctor; he immediately sent me to the hospital—I was in complete liver failure. I was in rough shape, with some sort of virus the doctors couldn't pinpoint, so I became determined to help myself heal. I read *The pH Miracle: Balance Your Diet, Reclaim Your Health* by Shelley Redford Young and Robert O. Young, and since I wasn't getting better in the hospital, elected to leave and do what I could to change the pH of my body from acid to alkaline.

I wish I could say I felt better right away, but I didn't. My liver enzymes got worse and everyone panicked. It took about three months for my liver enzymes to come down to a level where they were considered still high but less risky, but I'd known already that I was on the right track. When you're in liver failure you're not hungry. I knew I needed to cleanse my body, and not with the kind of diet I had been eating. I started drink-

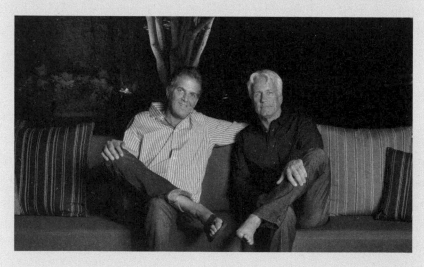

ing eight juices a day, all green, adding avocado to some of them for the fat I needed. I put in Brussels sprouts, hemp, and other vegetables and alkaline foods.

People who knew me thought I was insane. Before I got sick, believe me, I would have agreed with them.

My friends eventually quieted their criticism when they saw a guy who had been really sick come back from the brink of death, and they saw his eyes get clearer every day, and his mental acuity and physical strength return.

I was surprised that I didn't miss acidic foods or wine. I love red wine, but I have no desire to ever drink again. My liver can't take it, and I can't ever go back to that level of toxicity. And as much as I love living in New York City, big cities are toxic environments.

Your first line of defense should be the things that you put into your body. Food is medicine and medicine can taste good. Now I eat a lot of fruit, and a lot of salads. I still stay away from anything that's very acidic. I also stay away from sugar, grains, and refined carbohydrates as much as I can.

My entire way of thinking has shifted. What's important is taking care of your whole body, eating properly, exercising, trying to destress, having some form of spirituality, and living in a loving space. At the end of the day, it all comes down to common sense. You can eat a Twinkie for dessert or eat a piece of fruit or drink a smoothie. The choice is yours.

Hydration Helps You Lose Weight

The average adult needs to drink half their body weight in water every day. Your body is made of 70 percent water, and you need to nourish it with foods that are 70 percent water, too. That won't happen if you eat a lot of processed food containing loads of salt and chemicals, as these ingredients can cause rapid dehydration as well as high blood pressure. When you eat too much salt, your body retains water to get rid of the overstock of sodium that is pumping through your bloodstream. As a result, your heart has to work extra hard, and it causes your veins and arteries to constrict. The average person should limit their sodium per day to about 1,500 milligrams. That's only about three-fourths of a tea-spoon of salt. It isn't very much at all!

Many times you'll think you're hungry or have strong cravings for certain foods when you're not really hungry at all—you're thirsty be-cause you're dehydrated. And your brain can have trouble telling the difference. Next time you are hungry, do an experiment and drink some fresh spring water. If that doesn't fill you up, make a cup of hot tea. Still hungry? Go for a freshly made green juice. I guarantee after filling up on these three liquids, you will be satisfied until your next meal.

PHILIP'S STORY

I used to weigh more than four hundred pounds. I made every excuse there was.

I think I tried thirty different diets, and none of them worked, and I told myself that I'd just have to accept the fact that I was going to be fat my entire life. There are some people on TV who are obese like me and they're laughing and enjoying life, right? Maybe I can enjoy life like that, too. But then I realized that there had to be something better than not being able to fit in an airplane seat or being able to walk up a flight of stairs without thinking I would keel over. I started getting panic attacks. And then I reached the tipping point, and I turned it around. Literally overnight I stopped eating fast food and went 100 percent raw.

I lost 215 pounds and my old life. My new life is so much better. I am a successful life coach, motivational speaker, and author, and I help people change their lives as I did by helping them with my ten-day Get Juicy cleanse.

I used to eat thousands more calories a day. Now I basically eat about one-fifth of what I used to, but I am always full and satisfied and full of energy and vitality.

People believe they need sugar for energy, and we've become a na-tion of sugar addicts. My advice would be to switch to healthy sugars. When was the last time you made a fruit salad, with cherries and blue-berries and blackberries? Maybe put a little bit of honey on it if you're still craving something. Mix that all up and put cinnamon on it. Or if you need something as a snack, grab some figs or a few dates instead of a Snickers bar. After a while you can start to taper off the fruit and find the perfect balance with high amounts of greens, which is what I like to focus on.

It's not just about losing weight. I have friends who are fit and athletic, and they eat meat and potatoes and processed food. So I tell them that there's even more—after a cleanse they'll realize that their muscles recover faster, their sleep is deeper and easier, and their mental focus is a lot sharper despite the fact that they were already in amazing shape. That's what going raw can do for you.

I'd like to encourage you to take this challenge. The time will fly by and at the end of it you'll feel like a different person. The goal is to feel good and take care of your body. I finally figured that out, and it allows me to keep my weight off. I know you can do it, too!

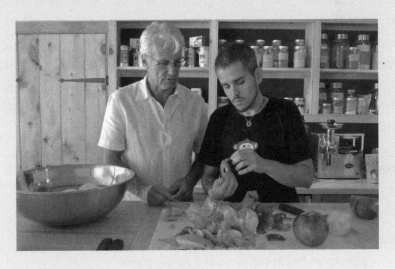

BETTER SKIN: THE MICRONUTRIENTS IN RAW FOOD ARE GREAT FOR YOUR SKIN

Along with weight loss and increased energy, you'll experience something else that will improve your appearance and attitude: You'll have a brand-new glow about you.

I told you my skin broke out when I first went raw. But then about three weeks into my raw-only diet, I was stunned to notice that not only had the blotches and pimples disappeared, but that my skin looked different. People who knew me told me I had a glow about me. Even the puffiness I'd always had around my eyes disappeared. And when I joined the raw community, the first thing I always noticed about a newbie to raw was the glow.

What's behind the glow? A detoxifying cleanse gets the gunk out—and since your skin is the largest organ in your body, it is going to show the effects of a good diet.

Once you go raw, you might soon notice, like me, that any puffiness or bloat you have had will start to diminish and then disappear. This is because a healthy digestive system not only eliminates solids from your intestines smoothly and quickly, but it gets the excess fluid out, too.

You should also notice that the whites of your eyes become clearer, your skin gets softer, your hair becomes shinier, and your nails grow stronger.

Once your skin starts to glow, so will your confidence. You'll start to feel better on the inside because the positive changes on the outside will be so wonderfully visible. You'll carry positive energy and a positive aura with you throughout the day. You'll have the glow!

MICRONUTRIENTS FOR SKIN HEALTH

Vitamin A: bok choy, broccoli, chestnuts, kale, pecans, pistachios, spinach, yellow and orange fruits and vegetables

Vitamin B: avocados, bananas, grapes, leafy green vegetables, nuts, pomegranates, seeds, sprouted whole grains

Vitamin C: broccoli, chard, citrus fruits, edamame, kale, peppers, strawberries

Vitamin D: You get this only from the sun; take a supplement if you are worried about too much sun exposure.

Vitamin E: almonds, avocados, blackberries, filberts, nectarines, peaches, pine nuts, pumpkin, olives and cold-pressed olive oil, spirulina, sprouted whole grains, sunflower seeds, Swiss chard

Iron: beets, leafy green vegetables, quinoa, soybeans, spinach, Swiss
  chard, turnip greens

Calcium: almonds, bok choy, broccoli, leafy green vegetables such as
  kale and Swiss chard, tahini

Magnesium: legumes, leafy green vegetables, nuts, seeds, sprouted
  whole grains

Zinc: pumpkin seeds, sunflower seeds

Selenium: Brazil nuts, oats, sunflower seeds, wheat germ

Biotin: almonds, cabbage, carrots, leafy green vegetables, onions,
  tomatoes

MICHELLE'S STORY

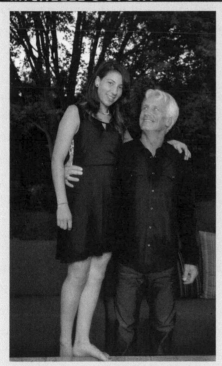

Brad is my uncle, and I learned about raw food from him. We had a family get-together and he brought these weird dehydrated things and everyone was saying how good they are, and at first I tried them and thought they were disgusting! But I don't think his kale chips are disgusting anymore. I love them!

When I eat raw, my skin clears up, my mind's not all cluttered, and I just feel better. So I like to spread the word. My roommates in Florida were always asking when a new shipment of chips was going to arrive. Another friend wants me to juice for her all the time. And it's fun because it's definitely a conversion once you get people to try it. They realize how delicious raw food can be, and it makes it a lot easier to start changing your diet.

BETTER SLEEP: YOU'LL BE MUCH MORE REFRESHED

I was not surprised when I read in a 2009 article published in *U.S. News and World Report* that nearly two-thirds of American adults say they are not getting the right amount of sleep each night. Even more shocking, according to IMS Health, a health care services company, Americans filled sixty million prescriptions for sleeping pills in 2011, up from forty-seven million in 2006.

I have taken a few sleeping pills, because I used to have my fair share of sleepless nights that led to very unpleasant days. I would have no trouble falling asleep, usually around 10 p.m., but I'd awaken at 2 a.m. without fail and not be able to fall back asleep for several hours.

At the time I figured that my insomnia had to do with stress, but I've since come to realize that while stress did play a part, the primary reason for my disrupted sleep was what I had been putting inside my body, like the big bowl of ice cream that I relished as an evening snack or my nightly glass of red wine, or the smoke or two right before bed.

I knew the unholy trinity of cigarettes, alcohol, and caffeine was doing me no good. I'd finally kicked my cigarette habit eight years prior to going raw, but it actually was harder to give up coffee and my nightly glass of red wine I loved so much. But I knew they had to go if I was going to stick to a 100 percent raw diet for an entire year, which I was determined to do.

Several weeks after my cleanse started, when the detox symptoms had completely disappeared, I suddenly realized that I wasn't waking up at 2 a.m. anymore. I slept solidly during the hours I was in bed, and woke up bright and early, with a calm and clear mind. What's more, I had boundless energy during the day. Let me just say that this was a very pleasant surprise, as I'd been an insomniac for years!

Once I realized how much my old diet had contributed to my sleep issues, I started researching raw foods that contained nutrients that are known to be sleep aids. Bananas contain tryptophan, the same amino acid found in turkey, as do almonds, sesame seeds, and sunflower seeds. According to the National Sleep Foundation, foods with a combination of a natural sugar content as well as tryptophan often help people feel sleepy. Pumpkin seeds help you drift off to deep sleep due to their high magnesium content; magnesium is a well-known and safe mind and muscle relaxant. If you have trouble sleeping, try eating a small amount of these foods before bed, as they should help.

I also incorporated a few other techniques into my life that helped me get more restful sleep. A few hours before bed, I switched to drinking water only, to make sure I was hydrated and that my digestive system would not have to work overtime. About an hour before bed, I turned off and unplugged all electronic devices, including my computer, phone, and iPad, so I would stop thinking about everything that was going on at work. Then I took some time to simply sit quietly. Some nights I would meditate for a bit, and other nights I'd just relax in a chair and enjoy the calm I was creating around me. When I listened to my body, it told my brain what it needed most.

Not only did my sleep improve, but so did my mood and my positive outlook on life in general. Much to my shock, I didn't miss my coffee habit. The only caffeine I consumed came in the form of green tea. Believe me, I never, ever thought I'd give up on wine, either, but I honestly didn't miss it at all for the entire year I cleansed!

JENN'S STORY

When I was a freelance makeup artist and also worked at a yoga studio, I would stop in my local café for lunch; one of their specialties is vegan raw food. My schedule was very flexible, and I was at a place in my life where I could pick up another job; they needed some extra help, so I started working there. Gradually, my diet began to shift, and as I stopped eating meat and upped my raw intake, I noticed that I felt better.

Now I try to eat clean. I don't necessarily eat raw all the way. If I can't, I don't. I don't stress it. I am lactose intolerant, and I do try to eat raw in the morning, like a smoothie and fruit. Plus I have a sensitive stomach, so sometimes in the evenings I'll lightly steam my food. The point is: If you're craving warm food, then eat warm food. Listen to your body.

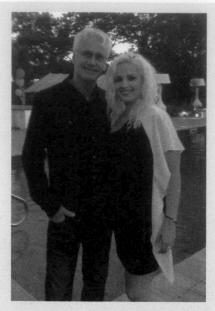

I noticed when I ate food like cooked meat, I didn't feel well and my yoga suffered. When I started eating more raw foods I felt lighter. I felt more energetic. I slept easier. Even my meditation changed—I felt more attuned to myself and more comfortable in my body, because my body was working properly.

Also, my skin improved, and my hair and nails grew faster. When I was in aesthetic school and still eating dairy my skin would break out and I had cystic acne. I had to cover it up and I knew that I was being judged by clients who wondered if I knew anything about skin care. But once I changed my diet and started using organic skin care products, everything changed.

My advice is to start small. Add juice to your diet. Don't be hard on yourself or upset with yourself if you eat something unhealthy—just be aware. You'll notice the difference and then soon you'll be saying, "This is a part of my life now."

BETTER BUDGET: YOUR SHOPPING WILL BE STREAMLINED

As you convert to your raw foods diet, you'll need to make a few changes in your grocery shopping habits. I've now gotten my shopping down to a science and am able to just run in for certain needed items. I've also saved myself literally thousands of dollars in food bills, because I don't eat packaged food anymore! It may take some getting used to, but it will happen for you, too.

As you dive into the meal plans in part 2, you'll notice that most of the recipes are family- and budget-friendly. A healthy raw food lifestyle should be easily accessible for you and your family, so I want to help you keep your food costs down. Note, though, that if you buy organic food the prices will be higher.

Nearly all the ingredients you'll see listed in the meal plans and recipes can be purchased at your local grocery store. If they're not available in your community, they can easily be ordered online through the resources listed on pages 251–252.

For tips on streamlining your shopping, see the section entitled "What should I know when I'm food shopping for my raw food meals?" on page 203 in chapter 9.

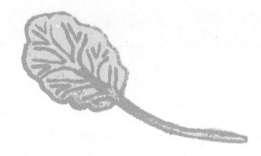

PART II
RAW MADE EASY

3

THE PLAN BASICS

B y following me on this journey you are doing something amazing for your body, and I am incredibly excited to share this path with you because you'll soon find out how easy it can be. Don't forget—I loved my steaks and red wine, but I was able to make this life change and I know you can, too.

I will introduce you to a world of green smoothies and juices that you make at home for yourself in less time than it takes to stand in line at the coffee shop. You do not need fancy equipment, and your home blender will work fine for the delicious juices, soups, smoothies, and salad dressings you'll be eating. A food processor will help with dips, salsas, and desserts. And although you'll see a few recipes for the dehydrator, it is by no means a necessary piece of equipment.

During the last two weeks of this cleanse you will transition into the 80/20 lifestyle, so I've included healthy cooked vegan dishes in the recipe section.

Once you have finished, of course, your 20 percent can be whatever you want. Do try, though, to eat 80 percent raw. The remaining 20 percent can focus on cooked foods that are, hopefully, primarily from plant-based sources, such as vegetables and whole grains. When you eat meat, dairy, or fish, look for items that are the best quality you can afford, free of hormones and antibiotics.

As you venture out and begin, remember that it's only 8 weeks. You can do anything you set your mind to for that time frame, and there are many powerful tools in this book to help you.

You will find sample pages for a food diary at the back. Use this as you see fit, but I have included questions to help you focus on the positives and keep you on track.

If you find yourself needing additional support, you can connect with me on my website. You will find more meal plans and recipe ideas on this site, and you'll be able to interact with other raw foodists through our community forums. Feel free to ask questions, as this is the best place to find the answers that will help you.

This chapter gives an overview of the Plan Basics. Please read it before you begin the plan, so you have a good idea about what you can expect. Chapters 4–6 provide menus and everything you need to know when you begin your transition to a healthy raw life.

AMY'S STORY

I joined the raw cleanse because I was curious as to what it was all about. I had known about the benefits of a plant-based diet for some time but I always ate a combination of cooked and raw foods, and I was curious about how difficult it would be to maintain this type of lifestyle. My preconceptions were that it would be very time consuming and that I would feel hungry and tired all the time. What I found was very different.

I will admit the first week was an adjustment; I felt a bit off for one or two days. After my body made the adjustment to an all-raw diet my foggy head cleared, and I was able to move through my day with a lot of energy. This was amazing to me because my schedule is packed! I am a mom, wife, and full-time high school science teacher. I am up at 5:15 a.m. every day and my first class starts at 7:30 a.m. Every hour I get a new set of thirty kids! I'm home by 3:45 p.m. to get my daughter off the bus, take care of household chores, spend time with my daughter, then schedule in a bit of time for my passion: health coaching! If the food I was eating on the raw diet did not supply the fuel I needed, I would have crashed; instead, I thrived. I found the foods actually easier to prepare than cooked dishes, and they were filling. I ate as much as I wanted and rarely felt hungry. I did not lose that much weight in the beginning but as the weeks went on I found my body looking better and feeling tighter. Toward the end of the cleanse I began to drop significant weight. Weight loss was not my motivation for joining but it was nice to see these effects.

I felt like the challenge pressed the "restart" button in my body. I realize how differently my body responds to different foods. As a teacher, I come in contact with many students and germs; I was on the cleanse during the flu season and I stayed healthy the whole time. I feel that my immune system was given a big boost!

My personal opinion is that everyone should do at least one 8-week raw food challenge or cleanse in their lifetime. Raw foods took me to the next level in terms of energy and vitality!

PHASE ONE: PREPARE (two weeks)

Rules for the Two Transition Weeks
- Focus on adding healthy, nutrient-dense foods to your diet while eliminating foods that aren't as good for you.
- Eat lots of salads and drink lots of smoothies.
- Wean yourself off caffeine, if you drink it.
- You might have times where you feel hungry, tired, or frustrated. These are all normal feelings and will pass. You will most likely feel fairly normal much of the time. This is a transition period to help you ease into raw, and the focus is on adding raw foods gradually, which helps minimize any potential side effects.

Week 1
- You'll add one green smoothie or juice to your breakfast every day. You can keep eating your regular breakfast, too, if you like. It's best to have your smoothie first thing in the morning, but if that's not feasible have it later in the day as a snack or with lunch or dinner.
- You should eat one salad every day. As with the green smoothie,

don't see this as a replacement, but as an addition to your regular lunch or dinner. Choose from the list of salad dressings in chapter 8, or use a dash of cold-pressed extra-virgin olive oil and Bragg apple cider vinegar.

Week 2

Focus on adding nutrient-dense foods to your diet while eating fewer less-nutrient-dense foods. You will start to eat some completely raw meals. This transition will set you up for success during the next four weeks.

For example:

- Monday: Green smoothie for breakfast only. At lunch or dinner add a salad in addition to your normal meal.
- Tuesday: Green smoothie with breakfast. Replace your lunch with a big green salad and have a normal dinner.
- Wednesday: Replace your breakfast with a green smoothie, have a normal lunch, and have a raw dinner.
- Thursday: Have a smoothie with your breakfast, replace your lunch with a big green salad, and have a regular dinner but add a raw soup.
- Friday: Have only a green smoothie for breakfast, have a salad with your lunch, have fun with dinner, and maybe choose something from the cooked vegan list.
- Saturday: Have a smoothie to replace breakfast, a raw lunch, and your normal dinner.
- Sunday: Last day of the transition. By this time you will have been eating so many nutrient-dense foods that your body will be craving them. You might not yet be aware of it, but your taste buds will start to change because your diet will have become so much cleaner. On this day, have a green smoothie with breakfast, eat your normal lunch, but have a raw dinner. Have something raw and scrumptious for dessert such as Mango Mousse (page 175) or Chia Chai Pudding (pages 175–176).

RAW OR NOT?

Food	Raw?*	Notes
Agave nectar		Read the label. Not all agave is created equal; some brands are boiled down at high temperatures to thicken the nectar. Look for a raw blue agave brand that is not heated above 115°F.
Beer	No	The process of making beer involves boiling prior to fermentation.
Chocolate		Read the label. Raw chocolate is labeled as such; other chocolate is melted above 115°F.
Coconut water		Read the label. Some brands use pasteurization, others do not.
Coconut yogurt	Yes	Coconut yogurt uses natural fermentation and no heat.
Coffee	No	Coffee beans are roasted above 115°F.
Cold-pressed oils	Yes	
Crackers	No	Unless it says raw on the packaging (meaning they've been dehydrated) you can be sure crackers are baked!
Dates	Yes	Most dates are sun-dried if they are marked "organic." Conventional dates are steamed to appear plumper.
Dried coconut	No	Dried coconut is often cooked. Sun-dried is acceptable.
Dried fruits	Yes	Look for dried fruit without added sugar. Some dried fruits are boiled in sugar water.
Dried vegetables	Yes	Read the label.
Fermented foods	Yes	Foods such as kimchi, pickles, sauerkraut, and tempeh use natural fermentation and do not use heat.
Fresh fruits	Yes	
Fresh herbs	Yes	
Fresh root vegetables	Yes	

Fresh sprouts	Yes	
Fresh vegetables	Yes	
Frozen fruits	Yes	Use frozen fruit with no added sugar.
Frozen vegetables	No	Most frozen vegetables are blanched prior to packaging.
Maple syrup	No	Although this is not a raw product you will see it used in moderation in many raw food recipes.
Mustard (stone ground)	Yes	Look for organic whole-ground mustard with no added salt.
Nuts	Yes	Look for nuts labeled "raw" and "organic," or for sprouted nuts that are then dehydrated.
Olives	No	Raw, unprocessed olives that have been sun-dried are hard, but not impossible, to find.
Packaged herbs and spices	No	
Powdered supplements	Yes	Read the label before buying.
Raw honey	Yes	If labeled "raw."
Raw milk	Yes	You can buy raw milk but it is not part of the raw cleanse.
Seaweeds	Yes	Most seaweeds are dried. Some nori is roasted to add flavor. Read the label before you buy.
Sorbet	No	Most commercial brands are pasteurized.
Spices (fresh)	Yes	
Sprouted grains	Yes	
Sprouted legumes	Yes	
Steak tartare	Yes	This is raw but not part of the raw cleanse.
Sashimi	Yes	This is raw but not part of the raw cleanse.
Sushi	Yes and no	The fish used in sushi is raw, but not part of the raw cleanse. The rice is cooked and can be part of your 20 percent once the cleanse is finished.

Tea	Yes	Many herbal teas are dried; there are teas that are roasted to enhance flavor. Read the label.
Vinegar	Yes	Look for organic vinegars with the "mother" (the substance containing the bacteria that turns wine or cider into vinegar) included—these are fermented naturally and contain abundant health benefits.
Wine	Yes	

* *Foods considered to be "raw" are those not heated over 115ºF. Foods that are roasted, blanched, or otherwise heat processed are not raw.*

PHASE TWO: SIMPLY RAW (four weeks)

Rules for the Simply Raw Weeks

- Eat 100 percent raw.
- Use the sample menus that are provided in the coming chapters. They will make your eating decisions that much easier.
- Use the recipes in chapter 8 and never hesitate to make your favorites over and over. Sometimes I enjoy the same green smoothie three days in a row.
- Plan ahead. Try to make some of the pâtés or dips on Sunday night so you have snacks ready to go in the fridge for your workweek. Buy a few packaged raw snacks to keep in the car in case you get hungry.
- If you are hungry, eat! This is not a "diet," so you should not be thinking at all about restricting your caloric intake here or starving yourself. You are focusing on eating good, healthy foods and filling up on greens.
- In the beginning, it is normal to feel run-down or tired, as if a cold or flu were coming on. Just blah and dragging. As the weeks go on you will start to feel lighter with an abundance of energy and an overall feeling of well-being.
- At the start of phase two, try to incorporate some of the lifestyle

techniques recommended in chapter 7. Commit to going out for a walk every day or journaling before bed each night. With this cleanse comes a chance for renewal, and it's not just for your body. It is also for your mind and spirit.

Week 3

The changes you made over the first two weeks should make the transition to eating 100 percent raw easy. Bear in mind that if you do experience any detox symptoms, they are likely to arrive during week 3.

- You will have a minimum of one green drink each day, either a juice or a smoothie. If you want to go crazy, have both!
- All your meals will be raw.
- Easy plan-ahead meals and snacks are included in chapter 8. For example: You can make the Raw Pad Thai (page 164) on Sunday night for dinner and eat the leftovers for lunch on Monday.
- Remember: If you are hungry, eat!

EASY AND FILLING SNACKS

These are some of the snacks I love:

- Any fibrous leafy green such as kale or spinach will be tasty and nutritious and extremely low in calories. Chop the leaves and serve a raw dressing on the side, which will make this snack even more delicious.
- Smoothies are filling and satisfying.
- Slice apples and dip them in raw almond butter.
- Grape tomatoes are as sweet as candy.
- Make your own trail mix. Combine your favorite nuts and seeds with raisins and superfoods such as cacao nibs and goji berries. This is a great snack to have with you on the road, but be sure to eat small portions, as trail mix is high in calories.
- Dates, bananas, walnuts, and avocados are very filling. Be careful, however, not to eat them in large quantities, as they are calorie dense.
- Health food stores have a large selection of high-quality packaged raw snacks. If you're looking for the crunch factor, you can buy raw

flaxseed crackers, raw leafy kale chips, and raw energy bars. You can even buy raw cookies and other sweet treats, but consume these in moderation, as they tend to be made with a lot of nuts and are often high in sugar. You can also find all of these products in my online store.

- When you're craving chocolate, you're in luck, as they are many terrific raw chocolate bars available in health food stores or online. Knowing that they can have chocolate has helped many people stay on the raw road for years.

WHAT TO SUBSTITUTE WHEN YOU HAVE CRAVINGS FOR SPECIFIC FOODS

For candy: Dried dates, raisins, plums, cranberries, apricots, and goji berries are foods (eat sparingly) that will satisfy your cravings for chewy, candy-like treats.

For ice cream: In a blender, place two peeled, chopped frozen bananas, ½ cup of almond milk, 1 teaspoon of vanilla, and ½ teaspoon of salt (optional). Blend until combined. Try adding 2 tablespoons of peanut butter for a rich creamy treat, or ¼ cup of cocoa powder.

For sorbet: Try 2 cups of frozen strawberries, 1 cup of fresh orange juice, and ½ mango. Pulse in a blender until combined. Eat as is, or place it in the freezer for 3–4 hours for a firmer texture. Experiment with other combinations of frozen fruit.

For pasta: Use a vegetable peeler or a spiralizer to make long peeled "noodles" from zucchini, summer squash, or cucumbers. Toss with your favorite herbs, fresh tomatoes, and a little olive oil.

For chocolate pudding: Mash a ripe banana with a splash of almond milk and a few tablespoons of cocoa powder. Top with fresh berries and enjoy.

For chips: Cut slices from large carrots at a diagonal and use them to scoop up some fresh raw guacamole or hummus. Munching on slices of colorful raw beets, jicama, or bell peppers also satisfies that need for a crunch.

For sweets: Slice a ripe piece of fruit, or have dried fruit mixed with nuts or a bowl of fruit with honey. Roll grapes in coconut sugar (found in health food stores) and freeze, or have a homemade Energy Bar (page 132).

For salty foods: Think celery, spinach, or sea vegetables, either as is or juiced. Rehydrate sea vegetables and add them to a salty spinach and celery salad.

For fatty comfort foods: Avocados or sprouted nuts are a quick fix. Or spread nut butter on your favorite fruit and top it with cacao nibs.

For warm foods: A dash of cayenne, red pepper flakes, horseradish, or a fresh jalapeño adds filling, satisfying heat. Or make tea, take a hot shower, or find a sunny spot to sit in.

For unknown cravings for something: Drink lots of water, and enhance it with citrus, fruits, mint, or even a slice of cucumber.

Other ways to curb cravings:

- Take a walk.
- Write in your journal—your own diary and especially your food journal.
- Meditate.
- Don't skip meals. Eating at the same time every day helps keep cravings at bay.
- Sleep if you can.

Week 4

You are continuing on your 100 percent raw path and by now are probably starting to get that raw and radiant skin glow! You might still feel some flu-like symptoms this week, but health benefits—such as increased mental clarity and better sleep patterns—will also kick in.

- Continue having at least one green drink per day. I encourage you to start your day with a green juice and have a green smoothie in the afternoon for a snack.
- Experiment with different lunches this week. Try wrapping your favorite guacamole and veggies in a collard green or romaine lettuce leaf. Really delicious!

- Make your own almond milk and add a dash of cinnamon, vanilla, or cacao for your sweet tooth.

Week 5

You may notice that you're losing weight. If you don't need to take off extra pounds, make sure to increase your intake of nuts, seeds, avocados, and oils. You should also notice improvement in your complexion, energy level, and moods. In fact, you'll be feeling so good that you should need no encouragement to keep going through the next two weeks. You'll find yourself craving your green drinks, and you'll look forward to creating a fun dessert to share with others. Don't tell them it's raw until after they have devoured the whole thing!

- Keep on drinking your green smoothies and/or juices every day.
- Add protein and superfoods such as spirulina and hemp seeds to your smoothies. You can learn more about superfoods in chapter 7.
- Meal planning becomes more and more important as your raw cleanse goes on. Although salads for lunch are typically the easiest route, experiment with something a bit more challenging. Make your lunch the night before so you are ready for the next day.

Week 6

This is the very last week of 100 percent raw! Time has flown by, hasn't it? By now your cleansing symptoms have most likely diminished, but if you're still feeling some of them don't be alarmed; the severity of the symptoms and how long they last depend on what your health was like before you started the cleanse.

You may be amazed at how much you are craving only healthy, whole foods and how you have integrated going raw into your lifestyle. You may even want to explore some more complex recipes. If you have a dehydrator, dive into the dehydrated recipes in chapter 8.

- Follow the rules in week 5, above.
- Check out the "Beyond the Meal Plan" self-care options in

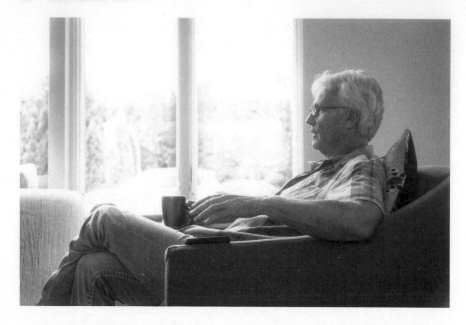

chapter 7. If you haven't already, do your best to start incorporating a few of them into your daily routine.

- Commit to a breathing exercise every day or go to the gym and try a new class.

PHASE THREE: LIVING IT! (two weeks and beyond)

Rules for the Two Lifestyle Weeks—and Beyond

- Be very proud of yourself, because you did it! At this point, you made it past what some might see as the hardest part (100 percent raw for thirty days). As you move into the maintenance part of the plan, it should be smooth sailing from here.
- Keep on eating 80 percent raw, and gradually reintroduce 20 percent cooked food into your meals.
- Try to keep the 20 percent as focused on healthy cooked vegan dishes as possible.
- You might feel more of the detox symptoms (achy, run-down) as you add in more of the healthier foods, but these should last

no longer than a few days. You might also still have some cravings for foods from your old diet, but they will slowly diminish as your eating habits improve. By the end of these two weeks, I predict you will experience a determined resolve to stick to this new lifestyle with a passion.

- Add more elements of the 80/20 lifestyle into your daily routine, which you'll read about in chapter 7.

Weeks 7 and 8

During both these weeks you'll continue to eat 80 percent raw foods. Let the sample menu plans in chapter 7 guide you.

- Continue having at least one green drink per day in the form of a juice or smoothie.
- Continue to eat raw for lunch or dinner. You can start to incorporate some cooked foods back into your diet in one of these meals.
- Figure that five of your meals per week will incorporate cooked foods. This allows for flexibility so you can plan around social and business events.
- Plan your meals in advance so you know which will be all raw, and which will incorporate cooked foods.

WHAT'S NEXT?

For maximum benefits after you complete the 8 weeks, I encourage you to try to stick to vegan/vegetarian meals for optimal health and wellness, but, of course, you can eat meat, fish, or dairy if you want to. If you eat meat, write it down in your food journal so you can be aware of what you've consumed.

My goal is to give you the tools you need so you know how easy it is to live the raw food lifestyle in a realistic and satisfying way. This is the plan I followed as a single guy with little to no equipment—I knew I had to make raw food easy and doable in my busy lifestyle or I wouldn't be able to stick to it. I was traveling when I first went raw and

I'd pack my blender in the car and go shopping after I checked into my hotel; that way I had no excuses not to stay on track.

Because I know how important it is to keep this lifestyle as practical and doable as possible, the recipes in chapter 8 were all developed to be accessible for everyone using ingredients from conventional grocery stores, and tested by Chef James Busch. Also, check the resources at the back of the book for online ordering. My mission is to make raw a reality for mainstream America. I know that if I can make the change, and stick to it, so can you.

In the next three chapters you'll find sample meal plans for the weeks ahead. Don't view this as a diet with restrictions. See it as the beginning of your brand-new way of life!

4

PHASE ONE: PREPARE

WEEK 1

Below you will find a sample menu plan for this week. Remember—this is just a sample. You can choose any juice, smoothie, or salad from the book that you would like to try.

This week is all about adding healthy greens to your diet. You need to have at least one green smoothie every day, either at breakfast or as a snack. You'll see on the meal plans below that some days include snacks, and some don't—this is up to you. If you're hungry, have a snack. If not, don't force yourself. You also need to incorporate salads as a side to at least one of your other meals. If you are feeling adventurous, replace your entire meal with a salad!

Don't forget to write down how you're feeling every day and which new foods you tried. You will be thankful you did when you look back to see the changes in yourself over the next 8 weeks.

Here's to a delicious week 1!

MONDAY

Upon waking:	Drink a tall glass of water and a hot herbal or green tea.*
Breakfast:	Arugula Ayurveda Smoothie (page 121).
Lunch:	Add a Caesar Salad (page 154) to your lunch.
Dinner:	Your normal meal.
Movement:	Take a thirty-minute brisk walk, optimally after a meal.
Journal:	Record what you ate and how you felt today.

*If you are weaning yourself off caffeine, as I recommend, gradually replace fully caffeinated coffee with decaf over the next two weeks, and drink that instead of or in addition to hot herbal or green tea. If you are using green tea, which normally contains a small amount of caffeine, to wean yourself off caffeine, then eight to twelve ounces once a day should do the trick. Then switch to fully decaffeinated green tea or herbal tea. You can drink as much of that during the day as you like.

TUESDAY

Upon Waking:	Drink a tall glass of water and a hot herbal or green tea.
Breakfast:	Brad's Green Smoothie (page 122).
Lunch:	Your normal meal.
Dinner:	Add the Dark Leafy Green Salad (page 156) with Baby Basil Dressing (page 147) as a side salad to your regular meal.
Movement:	Practice a breathing exercise.
Journal:	Record what you ate and how you felt today.

WEDNESDAY

Upon Waking:	Drink a tall glass of water and a hot herbal or green tea.
Breakfast:	Brad's Green Lemonade (page 125).
Lunch:	Brad's Favorite Seaweed Salad (page 155) in addition to your regular lunch.
Dinner:	Your regular dinner.
Movement:	Try a yoga class.
Journal:	Record what you ate and how you felt today.

THURSDAY

Upon Waking:	Drink a tall glass of water and a hot herbal or green tea.
Breakfast:	Enjoy your regular breakfast.
Lunch:	Everyday Raw Salad (page 154) with Grapefruit Star Dressing (page 149) in addition to your regular lunch.
Afternoon Snack:	Spinach Smoothie (page 121).
Dinner:	Enjoy your regular dinner.
Movement:	Take another brisk walk outdoors. Take a friend with you so you have a buddy!
Journal:	Record what you ate and how you felt today. It's been four days of extra greens and more movement. Do you have more energy? What is your mood like?

FRIDAY

Upon Waking:	Drink a tall glass of water and a hot herbal or green tea.
Breakfast:	Swiss Kiss Smoothie (page 120).
Lunch:	Have your regular lunch today.
Dinner:	Have your regular dinner tonight and add Fennel and Orange Salad (page 154).
Movement:	Maybe turn your walk into a thirty-minute light jog tonight.
Journal:	Record what you ate and how you felt today.

SATURDAY

Upon Waking:	Drink a tall glass of water and a hot herbal or green tea.
Breakfast:	Enjoy your normal breakfast.
Lunch:	If you are feeling up to it, enjoy Asian Coleslaw Salad (page 157) for lunch by itself. Otherwise, have it as a side to your regular lunch.
Afternoon Snack:	Señor Verde Smoothie (page 121).
Dinner:	Enjoy your normal dinner.
Movement:	Practice a breathing exercise.
Journal:	Record what you ate and how you felt today.

SUNDAY

Upon Waking:	Drink a tall glass of water and a hot herbal or green tea.
Breakfast:	Mean Green Juice (page 126).
Movement:	Look for an early morning yoga class in your area.
Lunch:	Enjoy your normal lunch.
Dinner:	Add the Tomato, Avocado, and Basil Salad (page 155) to your meal.
Journal:	It's the end of week 1! How do you feel? What differences have you noticed?

WEEK 2

You are still in transition mode: Week 1 gave you a good taste for what to expect, and in week 2 we are going to dive in further.

Continue to have your one green drink per day and incorporate more raw foods. Again, use the sample menu below as a guide, as you should always feel free to choose your favorites from the recipes. Enjoy!

MONDAY

Upon Waking:	Drink a tall glass of water and a hot herbal or green tea.
Breakfast:	Coco Mint Smoothie (page 122).
Lunch:	Replace your regular lunch with the Everyday Raw Salad (page 155) with Brad's House Dressing (page 146).
Dinner:	Enjoy your regular dinner.
Movement:	Do you belong to a gym? If not, check one out tonight. Look for classes such as spinning or Pilates.
Journal:	Record what you ate and how you felt today.

TUESDAY

Upon Waking:	Drink a tall glass of water and a hot herbal or green tea.
Breakfast:	Bloody Mary Juice (page 128).
Lunch:	Enjoy your regular lunch.
Dinner:	Replace your normal dinner with Dark Leafy Green Salad (page 156) with Sun-Dried Tomato and Kalamata Dressing (page 147).

Movement:	Incorporate a light jog into your evening tonight.
Journal:	Record what you ate and how you felt today.

WEDNESDAY

Upon Waking:	Drink a tall glass of water and a hot herbal or green tea.
Breakfast:	Brad's Green Smoothie (page 122).
Lunch:	Replace lunch with Deli Salad (page 156) over a bed of romaine lettuce leaves.
Dinner:	Enjoy your normal dinner.
Movement:	Head out to an evening yoga class. You are halfway through the week!
Journal:	Record what you ate and how you felt today.

THURSDAY

Upon Waking:	Drink a tall glass of water and a hot herbal or green tea.
Breakfast:	Green Vibrance Juice (page 126).
Lunch:	Replace lunch with Kolourful Kabobs (page 165). Prepare these the evening before.
Afternoon Snack:	Got a sweet tooth? Enjoy the Cherry Cacao Smoothie (page 123).
Dinner:	Have your normal dinner.
Movement:	Relax and focus on a breathing technique.
Journal:	Record what you ate and how you felt today. For example, are you having any cravings? Do you have more energy? Do you feel more refreshed?

FRIDAY

Upon Waking:	Drink a tall glass of water and a hot herbal or green tea.
Breakfast:	Arugula Ayurveda Smoothie (page 121).
Lunch:	Enjoy your normal lunch.
Dinner:	Brad's "Not So" Sushi Rolls (page 167).
Movement:	Take a brisk walk this evening. Maybe venture out a little longer than you have been used to.
Journal:	Record what you ate and how you felt today.

SATURDAY

Upon Waking:	Drink a tall glass of water and a hot herbal or green tea.
Breakfast:	Swiss Kiss Smoothie (page 120).
Movement:	Head over to your gym for a morning group exercise class.
Lunch:	Enjoy your normal lunch.
Dinner:	Raw Pad Thai (page 164).
Evening Snack:	Try some Chia Chai Pudding (pages 175–176).
Journal:	Record what you ate and how you felt today.

SUNDAY

This is your last day before you move to Phase Two and go 100 percent raw, so you're going to gear up with extra greens.

Upon Waking:	Drink a tall glass of water and a hot herbal or green tea.
Movement:	Go to an early morning yoga class to set your intention for the next 30 days of 100 percent raw.
Breakfast:	Kale with a Kick! Juice (page 127).
Lunch:	Enjoy your regular lunch.
Afternoon Snack:	Spinach Smoothie (page 121).
Dinner:	Everyday Raw Salad (page 154) with Brad's House Dressing (page 146).
Celebrate!:	Make yourself a Pineapple Basil Mocktail (page 129). Tomorrow your incredible journey starts.
Journal:	Record what you ate today and how you feel after the past two weeks. How do you anticipate the new month? Is there anything specific that you're thinking or wondering about?

5

PHASE TWO: SIMPLY RAW

Here we go! Let me assure you that the next four weeks are going to be amazing. Of course, it may not always feel easy to you since it's a major lifestyle shift, but you will be thankful in the end. Just as I was.

For the next four weeks, every meal you eat will be 100 percent raw. Look at this month as a learning experience and a time to experiment. You can choose from any of the recipes that are listed in chapter 8 with the exception of the vegan cooked recipes at the end (those are for phase three). If you find other raw recipes that you enjoy or would like to try, feel free to incorporate them.

You will notice some places where I include a snack midmorning or a snack in the afternoon. I vary them depending on the day, but do what works best for you. If you are hungry in the morning after breakfast have a snack then, even if the plan says in the afternoon. If you are hungry at odd times during the day, never hesitate to make a big green juice.

WEEK 3

MONDAY

Upon Waking:	Drink a tall glass of water and a hot herbal or green tea.
Breakfast:	Coco Mint Smoothie (page 122).
Morning Snack:	Piece of fruit or a fruit salad.
Lunch:	Dark Leafy Green Salad (page 156) with Baby Basil Dressing (page 147).
Afternoon Snack:	Watermelon, Pineapple, and Ginger Juice (page 129).
Dinner:	Portobello Burgers (pages 167–168).
Dessert:	Papaya Pudding (page 176).
Movement:	Incorporate at least forty-five minutes. Maybe go for a walk and do some light exercises at home.
Journal:	Take note of how you feel today. You are in for an amazing journey.

TUESDAY

Upon Waking:	Drink a tall glass of water and a hot herbal or green tea.
Breakfast:	Swiss Kiss Smoothie (page 120).
Lunch:	Everyday Raw Salad (page 154) with Creamy Green Dressing (page 149).
Afternoon Snack:	Banana Carob Smoothie (page 123).
Dinner:	Veggie Ribbon Noodles (page 166) with Marinara Sauce (page 153).
Movement:	Take a yoga class today.
Journal:	Record what you ate and how you felt today.

WEDNESDAY

Upon Waking:	Drink a tall glass of water and a hot herbal or green tea.
Breakfast:	Berry Smoothie (page 123).
Morning Snack:	Brad's Green Lemonade (page 125).
Lunch:	Brad's Favorite Seaweed Salad (page 155).
Dinner:	Kolourful Kabobs (page 165).

Dessert: Raw Chocolate Chip Cookies (pages 176–177).

Movement: Practice a breathing technique tonight.

Journal: Record what you ate and how you felt today.

THURSDAY

Upon Waking: Drink a tall glass of water and a hot herbal or green tea.

Breakfast: Collard and Pear Juice (page 125).

Morning Snack: Fruit salad.

Lunch: Hemp Seed Salad (page 158) with Greek Herb Lemon Dressing (page 150).

Dinner: Gazpacho (page 160) and Jicama Fries (page 139).

Dessert: Berry Smoothie (page 123).

Movement: Go for a walk outside.

Journal: Record what you ate and how you felt today.

FRIDAY

Upon Waking: Drink a tall glass of water and a hot herbal or green tea.

Breakfast: Green Vibrance Juice (page 126).

Morning Snack: Fruit salad.

Lunch: Carrot Salad (page 158).

Afternoon Snack: Peach Pump It Up Smoothie (page 124).

Dinner: Burritos (pages 162–163).

Celebrate: It's Friday Happy Hour! Have a glass of Champagne (page 130).

Movement: Go for a walk outside.

Journal: Record what you ate and how you felt today.

SATURDAY

Upon Waking: Drink a tall glass of water and a hot herbal or green tea.

Breakfast: Señor Verde Smoothie (page 121).

Lunch: Stuffed Mushrooms (page 166).

Afternoon Snack: Apple Pie Juice (page 128).

Dinner: Lasagna Rolls (page 165).

Dessert:	Brazil Nut Mylk Gone Wild! (page 172).
Movement:	Check out a class at the gym.
Journal:	Record what you ate and how you felt today.

SUNDAY

Upon Waking:	Drink a tall glass of water and a hot herbal or green tea.
Movement:	Take an early morning yoga class to set your intention for the following week.
Breakfast:	B8 Juice (page 126).
Morning Snack:	Fruit salad.
Lunch:	Zesty Kimchi (page 140) and South Pacific Oyster Mushrooms (page 163).
Afternoon Snack:	Green Seeds (page 138).
Dinner:	Brad's "Not So" Sushi Rolls (page 167).
Journal:	You completed an entire week of 100 percent raw— what an accomplishment! Even if you are feeling detox symptoms now, that's okay. Record how you feel and what you are looking forward to next week.

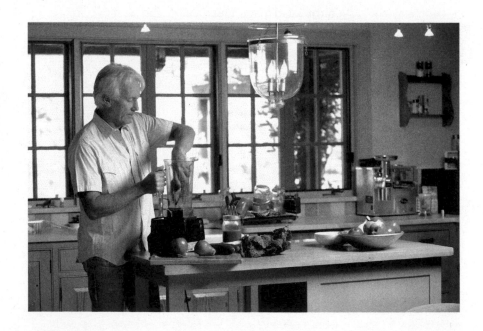

WEEK 4

MONDAY

Upon Waking:	Drink a tall glass of water and a hot herbal or green tea.
Breakfast:	Kale with a Kick! Juice (page 127). It is Monday, after all!
Lunch:	Your favorite green salad with Honey Mustard Dressing (page 150).
Afternoon Snack:	Peach Pump It Up Smoothie (page 124).
Dinner:	Corn Succotash (page 139) and South Pacific Oyster Mushrooms (left over from yesterday) (page 163).
Movement:	Take a class at the gym to get your blood pumping.
Journal:	Record what you ate and how you felt today.

TUESDAY

Upon Waking:	Drink a tall glass of water and a hot herbal or green tea.
Breakfast:	Cherry Cacao Smoothie (page 123).
Lunch:	Dark Leafy Green Salad (page 156) with Brad's House Dressing (page 146).
Afternoon Snack:	Cucumber Juice (page 127).
Dinner:	Veggie Ribbon Noodles (page 166) with Puttanesca Sauce (pages 151–152).
Movement:	Go out for a light jog tonight.
Journal:	Record what you ate and how you felt today.

WEDNESDAY

Upon Waking:	Drink a tall glass of water and a hot herbal or green tea.
Breakfast:	Señor Verde Smoothie (page 121).
Lunch:	Asian Coleslaw Salad (page 157).
Afternoon Snack:	Zesty Flax Crackers (page 135).
Dinner:	Portobello Burgers (pages 167–168) and Corn Succotash (page 139).
Dessert:	Tropical Gelato (pages 181–182).
Movement:	Take a yoga class and enjoy the night.
Journal:	Record what you ate and how you felt today.

THURSDAY

Upon Waking:	Drink a tall glass of water and a hot herbal or green tea.
Breakfast:	Papaya Pudding (page 176).
Lunch:	Cucumber Soup with Avocado and Dill (page 160).
Afternoon Snack:	Chocolate Fruit and Nut Bar (pages 172–173).
Dinner:	Stuffed Mushrooms (page 166) and Caesar Salad (page 154).
Movement:	Go out for a brisk forty-five-minute walk.
Journal:	Record what you ate and how you felt today.

FRIDAY

Upon Waking:	Drink a tall glass of water and a hot herbal or green tea.
Breakfast:	Banana Carob Smoothie (page 123).
Lunch:	Brad's Favorite Seaweed Salad (page 155).
Afternoon Snack:	Mini Fruit Bowls (page 170).
Dinner:	Kolourful Kabobs (page 165).
Dessert:	Green Vibrance Juice (page 126).
Movement:	Try a spin class—it's one of my favorites to get my heart rate pumping.
Journal:	Record what you ate and how you felt today.

SATURDAY

Upon Waking:	Drink a tall glass of water and a hot herbal or green tea.
Movement:	Take an early morning yoga class.
Breakfast:	Arugula Ayurveda Smoothie (page 121).
Lunch:	Brad's Raw Mac and Cheese (page 173).
Afternoon Snack:	Chive-Miso Flax Crackers (page 134).
Dinner:	Raw Pad Thai (page 164).
Dessert:	Chia Chai Pudding (pages 175–176).
Journal:	Record what you ate and how you felt today.

SUNDAY

Upon Waking:	Drink a tall glass of water and a hot herbal or green tea.
Breakfast:	Spinach Smoothie (page 121).
Lunch:	Everyday Raw Salad (page 154) with Thai Dream Dressing (pages 147–148).
Afternoon Snack:	Fudgsicles (page 174).
Dinner:	Zucchini Pizza (page 168).
Movement:	Practice a breathing technique and take time for yourself today. You are doing great!
Journal:	Record what you ate and how you felt today. You have been raw for two weeks! How do you feel? Is your skin glowing? I think it probably is.

WEEK 5

MONDAY

Upon Waking:	Drink a tall glass of water and a hot herbal or green tea.
Breakfast:	Coco Mint Smoothie (page 122).
Lunch:	Burritos (pages 162–163).
Afternoon Snack:	B8 Juice (page 126).
Dinner:	Lasagna Rolls (page 165).
Movement:	Go outside for a walk in nature.
Journal:	Record what you ate and how you felt today.

TUESDAY

Upon Waking:	Drink a tall glass of water and a hot herbal or green tea.
Breakfast:	Berry Smoothie (page 123).
Lunch:	Mayan Salad (page 159).
Afternoon Snack:	Mango Mousse (page 175).
Dinner:	Gazpacho (page 160) and your favorite salad.
Movement:	Take a class at the gym.
Journal:	Record what you ate and how you felt today.

WEDNESDAY

Upon Waking:	Drink a tall glass of water and a hot herbal or green tea.
Breakfast:	Bloody Mary Juice (page 128).
Lunch:	Easy Grated Salad (page 158) with Grapefruit Star Dressing (page 149).
Afternoon Snack:	Papaya Pudding (page 176).
Dinner:	Veggie Ribbon Noodles (page 166) with Pesto Sauce (page 152).
Dessert:	Brad's Frozen Green Smoothie Pops (page 173).
Movement:	Go out for a thirty-minute evening jog to get your heart pumping.
Journal:	Record what you ate and how you felt today.

THURSDAY

Upon Waking:	Drink a tall glass of water and a hot herbal or green tea.
Breakfast:	Brad's Green Smoothie (page 122).
Lunch:	Brad's Favorite Seaweed Salad (page 155).
Afternoon Snack:	Mini Fruit Bowls (page 170).
Dinner:	Brad's "Not So" Sushi Rolls (page 167).
Movement:	Take time for yourself tonight. Read a book or practice a breathing technique.
Journal:	Record what you ate and how you felt today.

FRIDAY

Upon Waking:	Drink a tall glass of water and a hot herbal or green tea.
Breakfast:	Cherry Cacao Smoothie (page 123).
Lunch:	Tomato, Avocado, and Basil Salad (page 155).
Afternoon Snack:	Brad's Rehydration Juice (page 129).
Dinner:	Portobello Burgers (pages 167–168) and Gazpacho (page 160).
Dessert:	Brazil Nut Mylk Gone Wild! (page 172) and Raw Chocolate Chip Cookies (pages 176–177).

Movement:	Go out for an evening yoga class to destress from the week.
Journal:	Record what you ate and how you felt today.

SATURDAY

Upon Waking:	Drink a tall glass of water and a hot herbal or green tea.
Breakfast:	Chia Chai Pudding (pages 175–176).
Lunch:	Gazpacho (page 160).
Afternoon Snack:	Raw Berry Crisp à la Brad (page 178).
Dinner:	BBQ Veggie Burgers (page 160) and Jicama Fries (page 139).
Celebrate:	It's the weekend! Have some Champagne (page 130)!
Movement:	Take a class at the gym or go for a run.
Journal:	Record what you ate and how you felt today.

SUNDAY

Upon Waking:	Drink a tall glass of water and a hot herbal or green tea.
Breakfast:	Eggplant Bacon (page 137) and Brad's Green Smoothie (page 122).
Lunch:	Deli Salad (page 156) over a bed of romaine lettuce.
Afternoon Snack:	Teriyaki Nori Crisps (page 171).
Dinner:	BLT (pages 163–164) and Jicama Fries (page 139).
Dessert:	Enjoy celebrating three weeks of raw tonight! How about a Raw Cupcake (pages 178–179)?
Movement:	Go for a walk today to clear your mind to refocus on the week.
Journal:	Record what you ate and how you felt today. Congratulations on completing three weeks of raw! Are you feeling the benefits? Are you experiencing better mental clarity? Document everything positive that is going on inside of you.

WEEK 6

MONDAY

Upon Waking:	Drink a tall glass of water and a hot herbal or green tea.
Breakfast:	Brad's Green Lemonade (page 125).
Lunch:	Asian Coleslaw Salad (page 157).
Afternoon Snack:	Green Seeds (page 138).
Dinner:	Fennel and Orange Salad (page 154).
Dessert:	Banana Carob Smoothie (page 123).
Movement:	Take a spinning class today. Really get your heart pumping!
Journal:	Record what you ate and how you felt today.

TUESDAY

Upon Waking:	Drink a tall glass of water and a hot herbal or green tea.
Breakfast:	Vitality Juice (page 128).
Morning Snack:	Mini Fruit Bowl (page 170).
Lunch:	Tomato, Avocado, and Basil Salad (page 155)—use a collard leaf as a wrap if you're in the mood for a sandwich.
Afternoon Snack:	Peach Pump It Up Smoothie (page 124).
Dinner:	Zesty Kimchi (page 140) and Everyday Raw Salad (page 154) with your favorite dressing.
Movement:	Go outside for a walk in nature.
Journal:	Record what you ate and how you felt today.

WEDNESDAY

Upon Waking:	Drink a tall glass of water and a hot herbal or green tea.
Breakfast:	Apple Pie Juice (pages 128–129).
Lunch:	Cucumber Soup with Avocado and Dill (page 160) and a small side salad of your choice.
Afternoon Snack:	Mean Green Juice (page 126).
Dinner:	Kolourful Kabobs (page 165).

Movement:	Take tonight for yourself. Practice a breathing technique and clear your mind.
Journal:	Record what you ate and how you felt today.

THURSDAY

Upon Waking:	Drink a tall glass of water and a hot herbal or green tea.
Breakfast:	Arugula Ayurveda Smoothie (page 121).
Lunch:	Dark Leafy Green Salad (page 156) with Miso Happy Dressing (page 148).
Afternoon Snack:	Grape-ade Juice (page 129).
Dinner:	Veggie Ribbon Noodles (page 166) with Macadamia Alfredo Sauce (page 152).
Movement:	Take a yoga class tonight and relax.
Journal:	Record what you ate and how you felt today.

FRIDAY

Upon Waking:	Drink a tall glass of water and a hot herbal or green tea.
Breakfast:	Raw Berry Crisp à la Brad (page 178).
Lunch:	Gazpacho (page 160) and Corn Succotash (page 139).
Afternoon Snack:	Pecan Spice Delight Cookies (page 180).
Dinner:	Burritos (pages 162–163).
Movement:	Go for a run this evening. Make it at least forty-five minutes.
Journal:	Record what you ate and how you felt today.

SATURDAY

Upon Waking:	Drink a tall glass of water and a hot herbal or green tea.
Movement:	Take an early morning yoga class.
Breakfast:	Papaya Pudding (page 176).
Lunch:	Brad's Favorite Seaweed Salad (page 155).
Afternoon Snack:	Sea Kale Chips (page 136).
Dinner:	Lasagna Rolls (page 165).
Journal:	Record what you ate and how you felt today.

SUNDAY

Upon Waking:	Drink a tall glass of water and a hot herbal or green tea.
Breakfast:	Eggplant Bacon (page 137) and Swiss Kiss Smoothie (page 120).
Lunch:	Zesty Kimchi (page 140) and leftover Brad's Favorite Seaweed Salad (page 120).
Afternoon Snack:	Miah's Energy Balls (pages 170–171).
Dinner:	Raw Pad Thai (page 164).
Celebrate:	It's really time to celebrate—four weeks of raw! Have a huge Mockarita (page 130).
Movement:	Go out for a walk today and reflect on the last four weeks of this incredible journey.
Journal:	You did it! You made it through an entire thirty-day raw food cleanse. Chances are you feel amazing. Write down how you feel. I want to know how you did. I'd love to see your comments on my community support forums.

6

PHASE THREE: LIVING IT!

Congratulations on coming this far! I hope you're feeling wonderful and you're craving only healthy and delicious foods.

You're now moving into the 80/20 portion of the plan. Since you have had six weeks to experiment with many of the raw food recipes in this book, the meal plans in this chapter are meant to help you navigate through the cooked foods listed at the end of chapter 8. Don't worry about sticking to exactly 20 percent cooked. Estimate and do your best. Remember to keep your raw percentage high and you will continue to feel amazing.

Try to stick to a plant-based diet for the next two weeks (and beyond) to complete your detox and help you achieve your health and wellness goals.

WEEK 7

MONDAY

Upon Waking:	Drink a tall glass of water and a hot herbal or green tea.
Breakfast:	Smoothie—your choice.
Lunch:	Salad and dressing—your choice.
Afternoon Snack:	Juice—your choice.
Dinner:	Raw dinner—your choice.
Movement:	Go out for a good run or a fast walk. Sweat out any remaining toxins that might be hanging out in your body.
Journal:	Record what you ate and how you felt today.

TUESDAY

Upon Waking:	Drink a tall glass of water and a hot herbal or green tea.
Breakfast:	Juice—your choice.
Lunch:	Miso Soup (pages 198–199).
Afternoon Snack:	Mini Fruit Bowls (page 170).
Dinner:	Raw dinner—your choice.
Movement:	Take a yoga class tonight.
Journal:	Record what you ate and how you felt today.

WEDNESDAY

Upon Waking:	Drink a tall glass of water and a hot herbal or green tea.
Breakfast:	Raw pudding—your choice.
Lunch:	Corn Succotash (page 139) and raw soup—your choice.
Afternoon Snack:	Cauliflower Popcorn (pages 142–143).
Dinner:	Spaghetti Squash Broccoli Alfredo (page 193).
Movement:	Get your heart pumping at the gym.
Journal:	Record what you ate and how you felt today.

THURSDAY

Upon Waking:	Drink a tall glass of water and a hot herbal or green tea.
Breakfast:	Smoothie—your choice.
Lunch:	Salad and dressing—your choice.
Afternoon Snack:	Hummus Fresco (pages 140–141) with veggies.
Dinner:	Raw dinner—your choice.
Movement:	Go out for a walk in nature.
Journal:	Record what you ate and how you felt today.

FRIDAY

Upon Waking:	Drink a tall glass of water and a hot herbal or green tea.
Breakfast:	Juice—your choice.
Lunch:	Raw soup and salad—your choice.
Afternoon Snack:	Superfood Apricot Bar (page 142).
Dinner:	Baked Artichoke Italiano (page 195).
Dessert:	Banana Carob Smoothie (page 123) or Cherry Cacao Smoothie (page 123).
Movement:	Go for a jog—make it forty-five minutes.
Journal:	Record what you ate and how you felt today.

SATURDAY

Upon Waking:	Drink a tall glass of water and a hot herbal or green tea.
Breakfast:	Juice—your choice.
Lunch:	Hearty Chili (pages 199–200).
Afternoon Snack:	Pâté Rosa (page 143) and veggies or flax crackers.
Dinner:	Raw dinner—your choice.
Movement:	Go out for a walk or jog.
Journal:	Record what you ate and how you felt today.

SUNDAY

Upon Waking:	Drink a tall glass of water and a hot herbal or green tea.
Movement:	Take an early morning yoga class.

Breakfast: Coconut Yogurt (page 131).

Lunch: Salad and dressing—your choice.

Afternoon Snack: Juice—your choice.

Dinner: Tempeh Holy Mole (pages 195–197).

Dessert: Mayan Chocolate Truffles (page 180).

Journal: Record what you ate and how you felt today. Do you feel different or notice any changes? Are you still feeling great? What do you think is the best percentage of raw/cooked for your diet?

WEEK 8

MONDAY

Upon Waking: Drink a tall glass of water and a hot herbal or green tea.

Breakfast: Smoothie—your choice.

Lunch: Salad and dressing—your choice.

Afternoon Snack: Hummus Fresco (pages 140–141) and veggies.

Dinner: Mediterranean Chickpea Stew (page 188).

Movement: Take a yoga class to start the week. Have you tried hot yoga yet?

Journal: Record what you ate and how you felt today.

TUESDAY

Upon Waking: Drink a tall glass of water and a hot herbal or green tea.

Breakfast: Juice—your choice.

Lunch: Salad and dressing—your choice.

Afternoon Snack: Smoothie—your choice.

Dinner: Thai Eggplant Curry (page 194).

Movement: Do some exercise during commercial breaks when you're watching TV.

Journal: Record what you ate and how you felt today.

WEDNESDAY

Upon Waking:	Drink a tall glass of water and a hot herbal or green tea.
Breakfast:	Raw pudding—your choice.
Lunch:	Raw soup and salad—your choice.
Afternoon Snack:	Juice—your choice.
Dinner:	Raw dinner—your choice (I love the Lasagna Rolls on page 165).
Dessert:	Raw Chocolate Chip Cookies (pages 176–177).
Movement:	Take today off to clear your mind and practice a breathing exercise.
Journal:	Record what you ate and how you felt today.

THURSDAY

Upon Waking:	Drink a tall glass of water and a hot herbal or green tea.
Breakfast:	Juice—your choice.
Lunch:	Truffled Mushroom Soup (pages 197–198) and salad—your choice.
Afternoon Snack:	Pâté Rosa (page 143) and veggies.
Dinner:	Your favorite raw dinner with a side of Zesty Kimchi (page 140).
Movement:	Go to the gym and get your heart pumping.
Journal:	Record what you ate and how you felt today.

FRIDAY

Upon Waking:	Drink a tall glass of water and a hot herbal or green tea.
Breakfast:	Smoothie—your choice.
Lunch:	Salad and flax crackers—your choice.
Afternoon Snack:	Mini Fruit Bowls (page 170).
Dinner:	Raw dinner—your choice.
Dessert:	Chocolate Mousse Pie (pages 182–183).
Movement:	Go out for a walk in nature.
Journal:	Record what you ate and how you felt today.

SATURDAY

Upon Waking:	Drink a tall glass of water and a hot herbal or green tea.
Breakfast:	Juice—your choice.
Morning Snack:	Mini Fruit Bowls (page 170).
Lunch:	Your favorite salad and Za'atar Almond Olive Pâté (page 143) with flax crackers—your choice.
Afternoon Snack:	Smoothie—your choice.
Dinner:	Black Bean Patties (pages 189–190) and Corn Succotash (page 139).
Dessert:	Butter Pecan Ice Cream (page 179).
Movement:	Take today for yourself and enjoy. You are nearing the end of this journey.
Journal:	Record what you ate and how you felt today.

SUNDAY

Upon Waking:	Drink a tall glass of water and a hot herbal or green tea.
Breakfast:	Juice—your choice.
Lunch:	Rawkin' Red Bell Pepper Soup (page 161) and salad—your choice.
Afternoon Snack:	Brad's Kickin' Guacamole (page 141) and flax crackers—your choice.
Dinner:	Oriental Stir-Fry (pages 193–194).
Celebrate:	Day 60! Have Lime Coconut Cheesecake (page 177) and a Pineapple Basil Mocktail (page 129).
Movement:	Go to the gym and get your sweat on. This is the last day of the plan, and hopefully you have a new outlook on life.
Journal:	Look back on the past 60 days. How was this process for you? How do you feel? Do you love this new lifestyle, and is it something you are going to stick with? Take time to craft some goals for your brand-new life.

BO MULLER-MOORE OF EATMOREKALE.COM

Q. Why did you sign up for the plan?

A. I was turning forty and my doctor was on me about losing weight and lowering my cholesterol and blood pressure. For years I was a picture of health, but age, kids, genetics, and life were catching up with me. My belly entered a room before I did; I began to feel like I was following my belly around.

Q. How did you feel before?

A. I felt chubby and slow. Frankly, as the "Eat More Kale" guy I began to feel a bit like a hypocrite. While I was eating plenty of kale, I was also eating plenty of everything else.

Q. How did you feel when you were working the plan?

A. To be honest, it was a challenge. Reining in my impulses took a lot of work and I was glad to be accountable to my health coaches at the Nourished Community. Learning how to shop and where to spend my time in the grocery store was key; it turns out I didn't have to take a single step into three-fourths of the aisles. I spent most of my time in the produce section.

Q. Once it was over, how did your diet/lifestyle change?

A. My diet will never be as it was before the plan. As I look back at the dough and grease that I ingested it makes me sad and sick. I now require a load of greens, veggies, and fruit in my daily diet. I make salads with lightly toasted nuts and homemade salad dressings that I crave. My smoothie blender is a blast, and now I could never live without one. These days I start every day with a big ol' fruit smoothie laced with kale. I do allow for a locavore carnivorous lunch, then a vegetarian dinner with no snacks after 8 p.m. I've joined the local gym and work out every other day for ninety minutes. I miss it if I miss a workout. I'm no purist or evangelical, but I have gained some self-control and perspective. That feels good, and feeling good . . . feels *real* good!

CONGRATULATIONS!—COMPLETING THE 8-WEEK PLAN

Congratulations on completing your 8-week plan!

I hope you feel an overwhelming sense of accomplishment for pushing yourself outside your comfort zone and allowing your body to experience the benefits of a cleanse. In the previous chapters, I've given you the basic tools you need in order to understand what raw is all about so you can continue on the path you've started. Knowing how to properly nourish yourself is crucial if you're going to move forward.

Many of the people I meet when I'm giving demonstrations or talking about my chips ask me if I am 100 percent raw—and you know, of course, that the answer is no. I follow an 80/20 diet and definitely do not deprive myself. Trust me on this—if, when I first started this diet, you would have told me I could never eat meat again, I sincerely doubt I could have gone through with it. But had I not embraced this diet, my entire life would be different. I would still be forty pounds overweight, sluggish, and not feeling well. It's highly unlikely that I would have created such a successful company or have been able to follow my passion and meet so many incredible people.

Here's how I live the 80/20 raw lifestyle:

- I eat raw foods 80 percent of the time. My focus is on a lot of green juices, teas, and smoothies, and I make sure to always have at least one green smoothie every day. I eat a lot of salads as well as collard green wraps and romaine lettuce boats. Because I am a single guy, living on my own and traveling constantly, I need to be able to make things that are quick and easy.
- For the other 20 percent of my diet, I really do eat whatever I want. I enjoy healthy vegetarian cooked foods. For example, some of my favorite dishes are the South Pacific Oyster Mushrooms (page 183) and sauteed hen of the woods (also called maitake) mushrooms. These mushrooms taste like steak and chicken, and they are incredibly satisfying. I also still enjoy meat every once in a while and sushi a bit more often. When I eat

meat, it is usually a steak, and now I always strive to find the best meat that is grass fed, organically raised, and hormone free. The restaurants I like to go to when I'm in the mood for a steak dinner—on special occasions; it's not a regular occurrence—serve only top-quality beef, and the chefs are always happy to discuss its origins with their patrons. I want to know where my meat is coming from. And I want to enjoy every bite of it!

As for eggs, I make sure that the chickens are vegetarian fed, free range, and hormone and antibiotic free. Same goes for dairy. If I'm craving some yogurt or cheese, I am always careful to buy it from a high-quality source where I know and understand the farming methods. Many supermarkets and natural food markets carry these products, and there's more information in the resources at the back of the book.

It is more than okay to question your farmers about their farming practices or question restaurants about where they purchase their meat and other food items. If they are passionate about providing the highest quality food, you will get a straight answer—and you'll probably make new friends in the process, because they will appreciate that you care and are searching for the best.

- No matter what I'm eating, I eat to enjoy food. I want to have a great meal with family and friends and make it an experience. It's not about eating on the run or scarfing down something from a plastic container with a plastic fork while standing in the kitchen (and yes, I have done this—or at least I used to!). It's about spending quality time with the people you care about and enjoying the moments and conversations that take place over a meal.

- I used to go on junk food and convenience food runs all the time. Now, "convenience" and "fast foods" are the smoothies I concoct every day. They take me only a few minutes to whip up, and all I have to do is pour one into a travel container and I'm ready to eat on the run if I have a super-busy day.

- When I do eat out or enjoy meat or dairy, I always wake up the next day and make a great big green drink, followed by a salad for lunch and lots more veggies for dinner. In other words, I eat just a little bit lighter, giving my digestive system a break and loading myself back up with good nutrients and potent enzymes.

BEYOND FOOD

In addition to eating wonderfully healthy and delicious foods, there are several other practices that keep me focused and feeling healthy from the inside out. I have come to not only enjoy but crave them. I'm going to give you my best tips for how I've chosen to live a plant-based and holistic lifestyle. I hope you'll find these guidelines for taking care of your body, mind, and spirit as helpful to you as they are to me. Believe me, if you'd asked me about any of them only a few years ago, I would have laughed. There's no way I could have envisioned myself doing yoga or meditating. So let me be the one to tell you that these simple steps can lead to enormous—and enormously empowering—changes in your life.

Find Support

I know I've said this already, but I was a single guy who lived the life of parties and big meals, and I was the last person who ever would have thought I was capable of completely changing my lifestyle. I am also the first person to admit that there is no way I could have done it on my own. I had incredible support, and one of the best lessons I learned when I went raw is that asking for help is not a sign of weakness but of strength.

Since I started my company, I have received countless emails asking me for help with transitioning to a raw lifestyle, and about how to achieve and maintain lasting success, so I created a health coaching and support system called the Nourished Community, which you can find by logging onto bradsrawfoods.com.

The Nourished Community is an online meal planning service; each Friday a new menu plan is posted with recipes and shopping lists. I know that eating raw involves more planning ahead than eating cooked food, and it is all too easy to get sidetracked when you don't have the proper ingredients in the house or when you get hungry. When your stomach is rumbling, it's much harder to make good food choices.

Included with the healthy meal planning service is access to community forums monitored by a team of health professionals where you can ask questions and seek support. You will find how-to videos and articles with the information you need to stay healthy. There's also a special plan section in the Nourished Community. It is not always easy to do this alone, and it's empowering to find raw food buddies around the country that are starting the challenge at the exact same time. You might even find someone nearby in your town that you can meet. (Check your local Meetup forums, too.) It always helps knowing there are others out there in pursuit of the same goals you are.

Wake Up Before the Sun Rises

I am typically up by 5 a.m., which helps me harness the energy of the day. I have a clear mind when I awaken. I like to start my day with a cup of hot green tea and then head out for a 6 a.m. yoga class or a workout at the gym. After my morning workout, I enjoy another cup of tea followed by a green juice or smoothie as soon as I arrive at the office around 7:30 a.m. I follow this schedule even when I am traveling on the road.

I'm not the only one who has realized the benefits of waking up early. The Ayurvedic philosophy states the importance of waking up twenty minutes before the sun rises. Ayurveda literally translates to "knowledge of life" and dates back five thousand years to ancient Sanskrit texts in India. This system of healing considers a person's physical constitution, emotional state of mind, and spiritual outlook, which Western medicine rarely takes into consideration.

I know that some people truly are night owls and have a hard time getting up in the morning. I have a friend who's a writer who can't focus before noon. Luckily, he has been able to fit his professional life to the rhythms of his body clock. So if your pattern is the opposite of mine, be sure to get moving as soon as you get up, no matter what time it is, then hydrate with a glass of water and some tea and then have a smoothie!

Harness the Energy of the Morning with a Meditation

When I first started exploring the raw food lifestyle, I realized there was much more to this cleanse than what I was putting in my body.

Early in my raw food transition, I decided to go on a ten-day vipassana meditation retreat. To this day I'm not quite sure what propelled me to do it—I only knew I needed to fill my spirit with good thoughts as I was filling my belly with good food.

For ten days, I did not talk to anyone, not even the staff members. I ate my meals in silence. I had no choice but to turn inward and get in touch with my true self, and I did this by meditating.

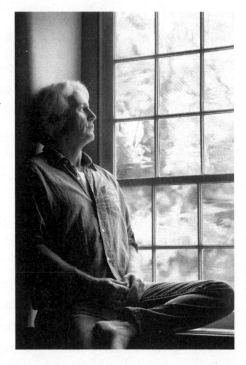

This experience of profound inner transformation is one of the most unforgettable events in my life, and I became determined to incorporate meditation into my life on a regular basis. It is my most important daily ritual.

Once my meditation is done for the day, I truly feel fresh and clear. No matter how hectic and crazy my day gets, I know I have taken time out to practice self care so that I can function to the best of my abilities. It is absolutely *not* selfish to say this. Everyone needs alone time—and the more demands you have in your life, the more crucial it is for you to try to find the time where you can help yourself feel good.

Why Meditation Works

Meditation is a state of hyper-awareness, and its purpose is to allow you to rest your mind and body—especially a mind that is stressed. It allows you to observe your way of thinking so that you can not only discover a solution to what is troubling you but also be able to redirect your attitude—move away from habitual and/or negative thought patterns and into a more positive outlook.

Every person will have a different reaction, experience, or outcome with meditating, but one thing I know for certain is that your mind will thank you for giving it a break!

I began meditating in my favorite yoga classes, but there are many other ways to begin. Take the approach that appeals to you—go to a meditation center, or use books, CDs, downloads, or videos.

Yoga and Why I Love It

Yoga isn't so much an exercise but more of a connection to life itself—at least that's how I see it!

I started stepping onto the mat when I moved back to Bucks County as a way to become more flexible. I was the kind of guy who didn't believe all the hype around yoga—I just needed to stretch out more and to try to shed some of the extra pounds I was carrying. As soon as I started, though, I quickly realized that flexibility and weight loss were the least of the benefits I was reaping from this practice. I became more physically flexible, but what was happening to me was much deeper than that. I became more open-minded and was able to control my emotions and reactions on a much deeper level. I learned that a lot of the poses I was practicing in class were helping to balance my hormones and unite my mind, body, and spirit.

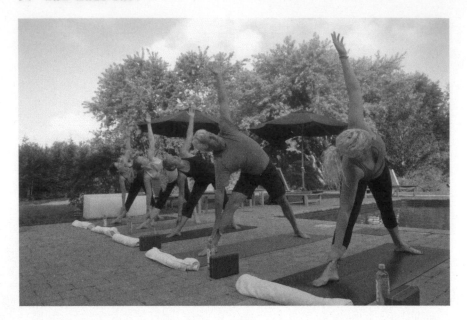

Many people from my past would be laughing at the thought of tough Brad Gruno making his way into yoga studios around the country, but that doesn't bother me. Yoga has changed me completely, and for the better. I have also found that many like-minded businesspeople, such as Jason Wachob, founder of the website mindbodygreen.com (my favorite resource for healthy living tips and the latest in yoga information), feel the same way about yoga as I do. Consider trying yoga, and I especially hope it will do for you what it's done for me.

ALEX'S STORY

I was raised a vegetarian, so I have a health-conscious background. If our family went to barbecues or birthday parties, my mom would pack our own food. When I went to college I was so busy it was really hard to eat well all the time, and I started to feel depleted. So I started juicing and learning about cleansing. Raw food just spoke to me. As a vegetarian it was such an easy transition.

I probably eat 98 percent raw, but I don't say that's the only way to be because what works for me might not be right for anybody else. If someone made quinoa and grilled some vegetables in coconut oil, what's wrong with that? It's nutritious and delicious and warming. The message about raw should never be that it's all or nothing. It's not.

And it's not about deprivation, either. A lot of people have said to me, "Oh, your diet was already restrictive, why would you restrict it more?" But I think what they're missing is that you're getting all of the nutrients that your body's asking for. Once you start really eating raw, you'll stop craving all those empty carbs or refined sugars because your body is fully nourished.

For me, eating raw also has a wonderful spiritual component. It grounds me and gives me a connection to my surroundings. I look at the world differently—it's providing me with all of these things growing around me that I need. I do truly believe that small things like just getting connected with the earth, and eating food that comes from the earth and that is good for you, can help you find a purpose. You'll find your thinking shifting from "I want to lose weight" to "This is the best thing for my health." It's been incredibly empowering for me.

Get Your Blood Flowing with Exercise

Exercising releases endorphins—your body's natural stress relievers, which is why runners talk about a "runner's high." You can experience these feel-good hormones yourself when you go for a hike, or walk, run, bike ride, dance, swim, or whatever you like. Getting the blood flowing is one of the best ways to improve your stress level and your health.

If you are new to diet and exercise, the easiest thing you can do is to start walking. If you're not in good physical condition, start slowly. The great thing about walking is that anyone can do it, and the more you walk, the more you want to walk. Get yourself outside in the fresh air and move yourself around.

I know a lot of people say they cannot find the time to exercise. Most lunch breaks today are at least thirty to sixty minutes long. If your break is thirty minutes, go for a fifteen-minute walk and drink your smoothie and eat a salad afterward. When you get home from work, try to go for another fifteen-minute walk (take the kids with you if possible).

Incorporating just thirty minutes of walking into your day will make a huge difference. Sometimes when I need to talk with my employees, we go out for a long walk; we're not only getting business accomplished but we're feeling good while doing so, and that helps us all make better decisions. We do this all year round, and even enjoy our walks in stormy weather. It's invigorating and puts everyone in a great mood (as long as their feet are dry!).

Even if you are feeling a bit crummy during the cleanse portion of the plan and don't have a lot of energy, try your best to push through the symptoms. Trust me on this: The worse you feel, the more you need to go outside and move around. The more you move and use your body, the more quickly your symptoms should fade. Consider this the next time you watch TV: The average hour-long program has approximately twenty-one minutes of commercials. Use the commercial breaks as a chance to get your blood flowing. On the first commercial break, do jumping jacks until your program comes back on; push-ups during the next break, then sit-ups, lunges or squats, or running in place. Before you know it you will have completed twenty minutes of exercise while watching your favorite show. If you can do this and still fit in a thirty-minute walk, that's nearly an hour of exercise. If you have kids, think carefully about what kind of role model you want to be for them. Don't be surprised if they want to join you for a walk or jumping jacks. I've included a Kids' Treats section of recipes in chapter 8 to help you make healthy, fun food with your kids. Now is the time to show them how to live the best life possible.

Relax and Release Your Tension

If you're like me, you might consider yourself to be a Type A personality—a person who takes on as many tasks as possible, fills your life with stress, and then works overtime to figure out how to get everything completed and under control. Even if this doesn't describe you, it's still important to take time out for yourself and incorporate some of these stress busters into your daily routine. We all need them!

Take Time to Breathe Deeply During the Day

Taking deep, relaxing breaths in your day will definitely help cleanse your system and your mind. Especially if you are feeling stressed out— and who isn't?

My favorite breath to take when I feel like I really need one is to breathe deep with my mouth closed, in through my nose and then out through my nose. As I exhale, I keep my mouth closed and make a loud, forceful exhale sound in the back of my throat. I repeat this breath a few times each day, especially when I start to feel stress catching up with me.

Take breaths like this during your morning shower, when your back is to the water flow, and each time you are stopped at a red light throughout the day. The more you practice this breath, the more your lungs will expand, pushing more oxygen into your blood and giving you more energy during the day.

Turn Off Your Electronic Devices

I run most of my business from my computer, iPad, and iPhone. There is hardly a minute in my day where you will see me detached from these devices. The only way I can tear myself away from the glowing screens is to put these devices away, out of sight. Otherwise, it's impossible to wind down and relax.

There are times when I will even turn my phone off for an hour. Having some quiet time away from these electronics and allowing myself time to practice breath work is one of my favorite ways to relieve stress!

Quiet Time Alone

I love to be social and visit friends and family, but when I go home at night to my barn, it's nice to have some quiet time to myself. On the weekends, I enjoy quiet time by mowing the lawn on the property with the riding mower. It's like a moving meditation. I get to be outside, in peace, and the yard looks terrific!

Massage/Reiki

Getting massages helps me deal with stress. I realize massage can be expensive and treatments aren't always accessible to everyone, but if you can, try to get at least one massage during these 8 weeks—even if it's the only one you do all year. It will definitely help you feel a bit pampered. You deserve it.

Use Essential Oils

Aromatherapy is the use of scented essential oils to improve your mood and boost your health. Basil, chamomile, and lavender are well-known calmers. Put a touch of lavender on your wrists in the morning or your sheets at night; you will feel your mood improve in a matter of minutes!

Take a Nap

I know this is easier said than done, but taking even a fifteen-minute power nap has been proven to help increase productivity and reset your mind. According to a 2008 poll by the National Sleep Foundation, 28 percent of 1,000 respondents said sleepiness interferes with their daytime activities at least a few days each month. If this happens to you, find a place where you can close your eyes and rest for fifteen minutes. Try using earplugs and a sleep mask if there is a lot of ambient noise or light. You might be surprised at how stress relieving this can be. (Just be sure not to oversleep!)

Wind Down for the Night and Then Get Enough Sleep

Without proper rest for your mind and body, you can't ever function at your optimal level. If winding down and getting a good night's sleep is hard for you to do, I hope some of these nighttime rituals will help.

Take a Hot Shower or Bath

Taking a hot shower or bath at the end of the day is a great way to calm down. Let the steam build in the shower, and practice your breathing. Light a candle in a safe place in the bathroom and find a way to separate your mind from the day's activities. Take this time out for yourself, especially if you have a busy family life. Your partner can watch the kids for a few minutes!

No Electronics an Hour Before Bed

You might like to fall asleep with the TV on, but it's time for that habit to stop. Turn off the TV, your computer, your iPad, and your phone at least an hour before bed. Can't turn off your phone? (I have a hard time doing that, too.) At least put it on silent or vibrate so you are not interrupted in the evening by notifications and messages. There's no way you can start to unwind if you're concentrating on your messages and not yourself.

Drink Decaffeinated Organic Tea

Drinking tea before bed has become one of my favorite rituals. Pick an herbal tea you enjoy and sip it before bedtime. It will calm you down and make you feel wonderful. Not in the mood for tea? That's okay—just heat up some water and squeeze some fresh lemon in it. If you are in the mood for a sweet, add a dash of honey.

Refrain from Eating at Least Two Hours Before Bed

This can be hard, depending on your schedule, but try your best to take the time to finish your meals at least two hours before bedtime. Going to bed on a full stomach might keep you up at night; you can't fully relax while your body is busy digesting all that food. If you need to eat late at night because of your schedule, though, opt for something light such as a smoothie, soup, or juice.

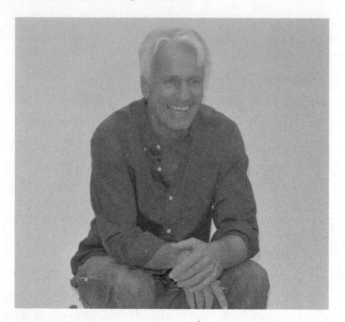

Start a Three-Blessings Journal

Right before bed, jot down three things that you are grateful for, or three things about your day that made you feel blessed. Writing them down will help reset your focus and your mind to take away some of your stress. It is also nice to look back on over time and remember all the good things that have happened to you. Keeping this journal and using it to visualize things that you have been blessed with is an amazing way to release natural endorphins, too.

Use a White Noise Machine or the Sleep Machine App

If you are still having a hard time falling asleep at night, try using a white noise machine that plays rhythmic sounds such as rainfall, wind, beach waves, or white noise, or downloading a phone app called Sleep Machine, which is programmed to play these rhythmic sounds. I know I said no electronics, but these devices can help lull you to sleep.

7

PLANNING FOR SUCCESS—THE ESSENTIAL INGREDIENTS

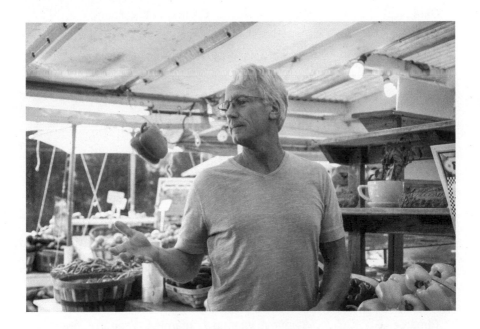

I n this chapter you'll find information about the most nutritionally dense vegetables, legumes, fruit, seeds, grains, oils, and sweeteners. Include as many of these as possible in your meals every day.

VEGETABLES	GOOD SOURCE OF THESE NUTRIENTS
Arugula	Vitamin B$_6$, copper, riboflavin, thiamin, zinc
Asparagus	Calcium, magnesium, pantothenic acid, selenium, zinc
Bell peppers	Vitamin C
Broccoli	Vitamin A, vitamin C, vitamin K
Brussels sprouts	Vitamin C, vitamin K

Carrots	Vitamin A, vitamin C, vitamin K, potassium
Cauliflower	Vitamin B$_6$, vitamin C, vitamin K, folate
Green cabbage	Vitamin C, vitamin K, calcium, manganese
Green onion	Vitamin A, vitamin B$_6$, vitamin C, manganese, potassium
Mustard greens	Vitamin A, vitamin C, calcium, manganese
Okra	Vitamin A, vitamin C, vitamin K, calcium, magnesium, manganese
Peas	Vitamin A, vitamin C, vitamin K, folate, iron, phosphorus, thiamin
Red cabbage	Vitamin A, vitamin C, vitamin K, manganese
Red onions	Vitamin B$_6$, vitamin C, manganese
Red potatoes	Vitamin B$_6$, vitamin C, folate, niacin
Romaine lettuce	Vitamin A, vitamin K
Spinach	Vitamin A, vitamin C, vitamin K, folate, iron, magnesium, manganese
Summer squash	Vitamin A, vitamin B$_6$, vitamin C, manganese, potassium
Sweet potatoes	Vitamin A, vitamin B$_6$, copper, fiber, manganese, pantothenic acid, potassium
Tomatoes	Vitamin A, vitamin C, vitamin E, vitamin K, fiber, potassium
Zucchini	Vitamin B$_6$, vitamin C, vitamin K, fiber, folate, riboflavin

LEGUMES	GOOD SOURCE OF THESE NUTRIENTS

Sprouted legumes are an excellent way to get protein and fiber.

Adzuki beans	Copper, fiber, folate, iron, manganese, niacin, phosphorus, potassium, protein, thiamin, zinc
Black beans	Fiber, folate, magnesium, phosphorus, potassium, protein, thiamin
Butter beans	Vitamin A, vitamin C, protein, riboflavin, thiamin

Great northern beans	Fiber, folate, magnesium, protein
Green beans	Vitamin B$_6$, vitamin C, copper, fiber, niacin
Kidney beans	Fiber, iron, protein, thiamin
Lentils	Fiber, iron, manganese, phosphorus, protein, thiamin
Lima beans	Fiber, iron, protein
Mung beans	Calcium, folate, iron, protein
Pinto beans	Vitamin B$_6$, fiber, niacin, protein, riboflavin
Red kidney beans	Vitamin C, fiber, iron, protein

FRUITS	GOOD SOURCE OF THESE NUTRIENTS
Acai berries	Antioxidants, beneficial omega-9 and omega-6 fatty acids
Apples	Vitamin C, fiber
Apricots	Vitamin A, vitamin C
Avocados	Vitamin B complex, vitamin E, vitamin K, monounsaturated fat, potassium
Bananas	Vitamin C, fiber, manganese, potassium
Blueberries	Vitamin C, vitamin K, fiber
Cantaloupe	Vitamin A, vitamin B$_6$, vitamin C, fiber, folate, niacin, potassium
Cherries	Vitamin C, fiber, potassium
Cranberries	Vitamin C, vitamin E, vitamin K, fiber, manganese
Raisins	Vitamin B$_6$, calcium, copper, fiber, manganese, iron, riboflavin, thiamin
Raspberries	Vitamin C, fiber, manganese
Strawberries	Vitamin C, fiber, folate, manganese
Watermelon	Vitamin A, vitamin C

NUTS AND SEEDS   GOOD SOURCE OF THESE NUTRIENTS

Making your own nut milks is cheaper than buying them. Find instructions on page 124.

Almonds	Vitamin E, calcium
Brazil nuts	Copper, phosphorus, selenium
Cashews	Calcium, copper, iron, magnesium, manganese, phosphorus
Chia seeds	Antioxidants, beneficial omega-3 and omega-6 fatty acids, protein
Filberts	Vitamin E, copper, iron, manganese
Flaxseeds	Beneficial omega-3 fatty acids
Hazelnuts	Vitamin E, copper, manganese
Pecans	Fiber, manganese
Pine nuts	Iron, manganese
Pistachios	Vitamin B_6, copper, iron, thiamin
Pumpkin seeds	Vitamin K, copper, iron, protein, zinc
Sesame seeds	Calcium, iron
Sunflower seeds	Vitamin B_6, copper, magnesium, phosphorous, thiamin
Walnuts	Beneficial omega-3 fatty acids, copper, manganese, protein

GRAINS   GOOD SOURCE OF THESE NUTRIENTS

Sprouting grains makes the nutrients more available to your body and the grains easier to digest.

Amaranth	Vitamin A, vitamin C, folate
Barley	Fiber, iron, manganese
Brown rice	Fiber, manganese, selenium
Bulgur	Fiber, iron, magnesium, manganese
Millet	Iron, manganese

Oats	Fiber, iron, thiamin
Quinoa	Folate, iron, magnesium, phosphorus, protein
Spelt	Fiber, iron, manganese, phosphorus
Wheat berries	Magnesium, manganese, selenium

SUPERFOODS

The term "superfood" is used to describe foods that are high in phytochemicals and beneficial nutrients and low in calories and fat. Not only are they good for you, but they also taste delicious! Many superfoods have antioxidant properties, help strengthen the immune system, decrease inflammation, and have antiaging properties. Plus, many superfoods come in powder form, so it's easy to add them to your smoothies and salad dressings for an extra burst of flavor and energy.

Goji Berries

Goji berries grow on an evergreen shrub native to Asia and Europe. Small and oblong, they range in color from light yellow to dark orange to deep rosy red, with a chewy texture and sweet-tart taste. In health food stores you'll generally find the dark orange and red variety. Goji berries are adaptogens, meaning they help invigorate and strengthen the adrenal glands, which help our bodies deal with stress. They are loaded with antioxidants; are an excellent source of protein; and contain a slew of trace minerals such as copper, iron, zinc, calcium, germanium, phosphorus, and selenium, as well as vitamins B_1, B_2, B_6, and E.

Cacao

Many chocolate lovers are familiar with this superfood already, but did you know that it offers one of the highest concentrations of antioxidants of any known food? Antioxidants help protect us from age-related health conditions, as well as from free-radical damage. Cacao is loaded with minerals such as magnesium, iron, chromium, manganese, zinc, and copper, as well as vitamin C and omega-6 fatty acids.

Maca

Maca is a root that is cultivated in the Peruvian Andes of South America. Like goji berries, it is an adaptogen and builds resistance against chemical, biological, or bodily stresses. It is said to help with anemia, fatigue, menstruation discomfort, bad memory, and tension. It also increases oxygen levels in the blood, which is especially useful if you live in or are traveling to a high-altitude destination. You can find maca in your health food store sold in a powder form. It's an ideal addition to smoothies and other drinks.

Raw Honey

Unfiltered raw honey is loaded with minerals, enzymes, and antioxidants. It also has antifungal, antibiotic, and antiviral properties, which is why different civilizations over the centuries have used it to treat and heal surface wounds. When taken internally, honey has been shown to provide relief from ulcers, upset stomachs, irritable bowel syndrome, and staph infections.

Bee Pollen

Bee pollen contains vitamin B_9 and all twenty-two amino acids. It is high in protein, contains antioxidants, is an excellent energy source, and helps your body recover after exercise.

Spirulina

Spirulina is a blue-green algae that grows in various lakes and waterways all over the world. It is green due to its chlorophyll content, and blue from a pigment called phycocyanin. Spirulina contains a vast array

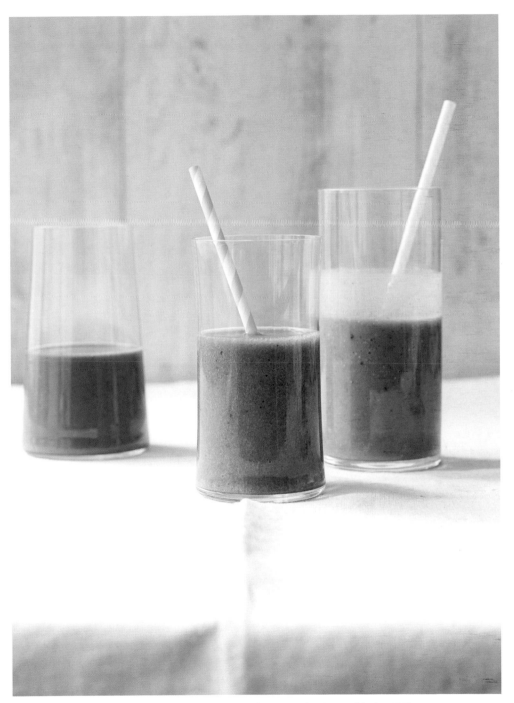

Brad's Green Smoothie (p. 122), Coco Mint Smoothie (p. 122),
Peach Pump It Up Smoothie (p. 124)

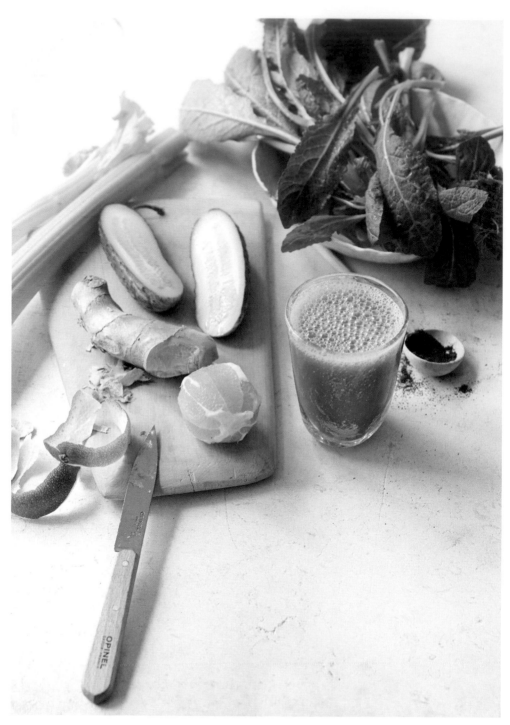

Brad's Wake-Up Juice (p. 127)

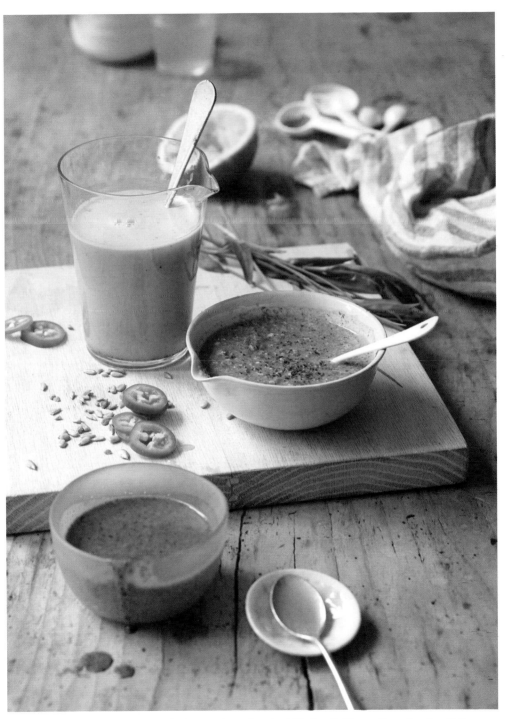

Clockwise from top: Grapefruit Star Dressing (p. 149), Brad's House Dressing (p. 146),
Creamy Green Dressing (p. 149)

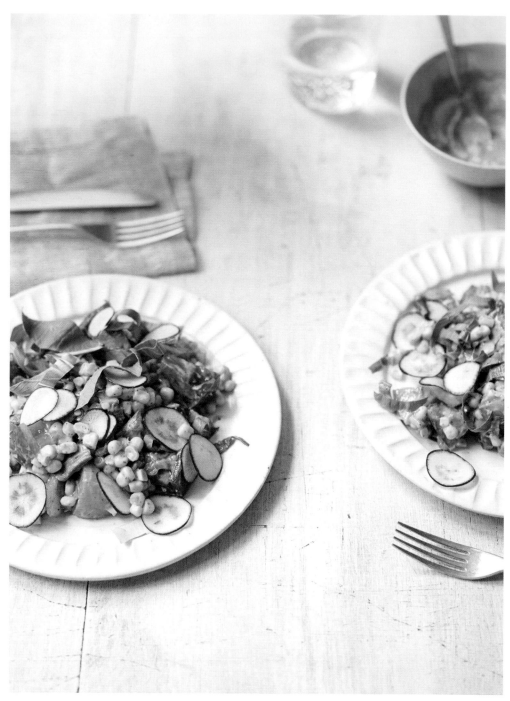

Mayan Salad (p. 159)

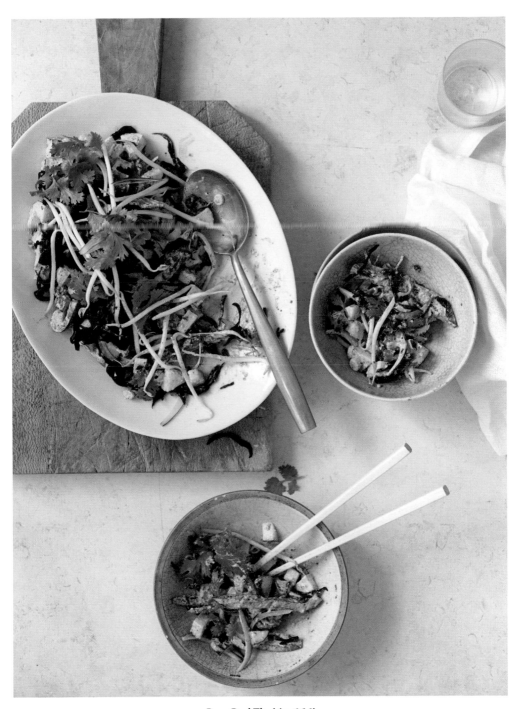

Raw Pad Thai (p. 164)

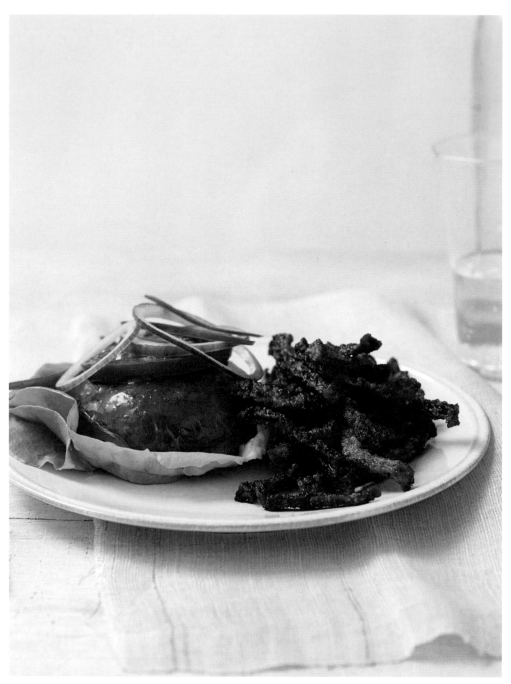

Portobello Burger (p. 167) with Jicama Fries (p. 139)

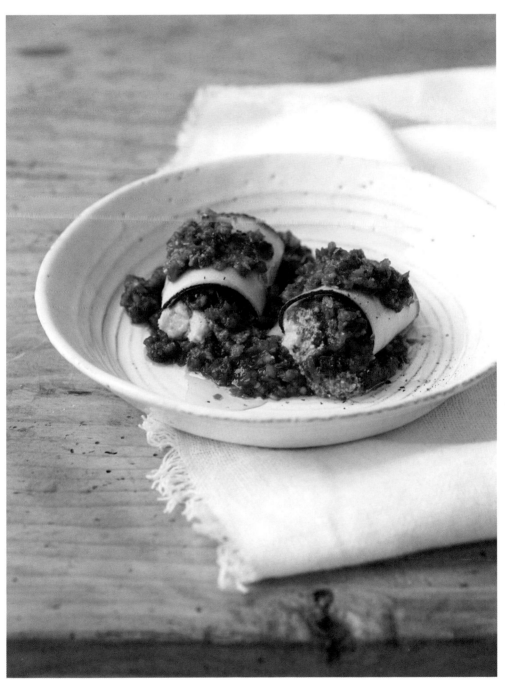

Lasagna Rolls (p. 165)

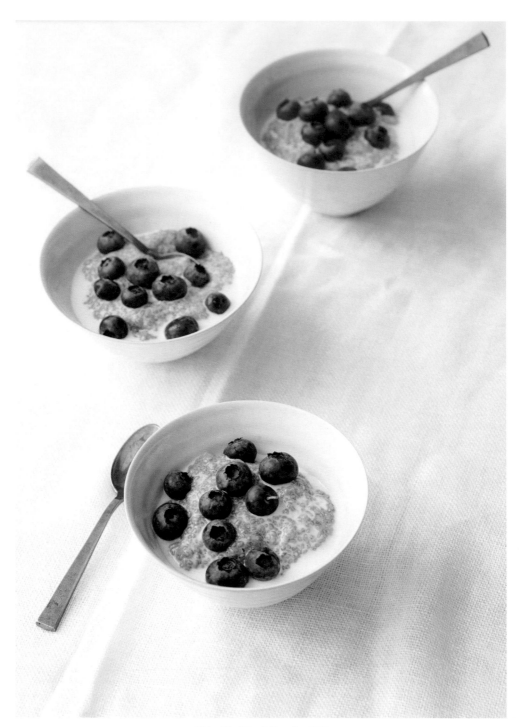

Chia Chai Pudding (p. 175)

of antioxidants, nutrients, trace minerals, vitamins, chlorophyll, protein (10 grams provides 7 grams of protein!), nucleic acids, and vitamins A, B_1, B_2, B_6, E, and K. It has also been shown to help increase the amount of antibodies in your immune system, which is handy when you feel a cold coming on.

Seaweed

Seaweed is incredibly nutritious, as it has access to and absorbs nutrients found in seawater. It contains iodine, an essential trace element needed by your thyroid gland to regulate your metabolism, is very high in calcium, and helps regulate, purify, and alkalinize your bloodstream. It also contains the nine essential amino acids and is easily digestible. Many different types of seaweed are found in most health food stores; the most common are nori, dulse, kelp, arame, and wakame. Remember that if the seaweed is roasted, it is no longer raw.

DANIELA'S STORY

Q. When did you start thinking about raw food?

A. I used to be really hungry all of the time, probably because I wasn't getting any nutrients and my body was craving them. When I started drinking raw juices I lost ten pounds and I was never hungry. I felt really different—not lethargic at all. I went to the health food store and pretty much bought everything I didn't know about and started experimenting. And when I decided that I wanted to create my own restaurant concept, with a juice bar and café, I opened Zia's Restaurant in Towson, Maryland, in 2005.

Q. How did you devise your menu?

A. Basically, my customers were the ones who guided me into raw food, through their requests. My grandmother, who was eighty years old, was there with me every single day when I opened the restaurant, and she worked on recipes with me. The more we worked on raw food, the more I realized that I had found my creative soul in the kitchen.

Q. What do you think is the biggest misperception about eating raw foods?

A. That you're not going to get protein and nutrients. And that the food won't taste good. But if you eat a ripe tomato right from the garden, how can it not taste good?

Q. How do you advise newbies to raw to start?

A. Salads are the way to go. They don't have to be salads with lettuce; I'm a big fan of something that has some heft to it, like a Turkish chopped salad, with peppers and onions and tomatoes.

Make sure you're getting enough fat—don't worry about the calories, especially if you're eating a lot of greens. You don't need a lot of fancy equipment. Even if you're not a chef you can create delicious dishes once you learn the basics. It's very easy to figure out that when you soak cashews and blend them they turn into a cream, or that adding coconut oil to raw desserts will allow them to harden when you leave them to set in the fridge, just like Jell-O. If you overcook things, they're often inedible. You're never going to have to worry about overcooking raw food!

Q. How about managing a sugar addiction?

A. Losing your taste for sugar can take a long time. You can eat raw food and still have a sugar addiction—dates, fruit, maple syrup, agave, and honey are all sweeteners. But once you adjust to eating a really clean diet for a long time, you're not going to crave sugar. I confess that I used to have a candy drawer at my bedside table; sugar was my drug. And I totally lost my taste for it when I started eating raw. I feel so much better, emotionally and physically, without it.

Q. Do you like smoothies?

A. I'm not a smoothie lover but my boyfriend is. People often tout the value of smoothies, but if you don't like them, don't make them.

I make my boyfriend smoothies with raw cacao, maca, goji berries, a little banana, some bee pollen, and raw honey. It's very sweet and milkshake-like, and I am gradually tapering down the sugar content. I

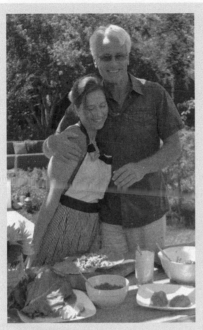

did try to sneak in some kale but he detected it. I'm going to have to go one leaf at a time.

Q. That's a great philosophy: one leaf at a time! Why do you think people are so disconnected from food?
A. When I visit my family in Italy, we cook all day long. We go to the market and pick up food and then make meals together as a family. We don't do that here in the United States. We're not teaching our children how to cook and we're not eating together, either. My advice is to try using raw food as a way to bring your family to eat at the family table, especially by getting everybody to make something together that they enjoy.

FERMENTED FOODS

Fermented foods are those that have begun to be broken down by organic acids, bacteria, and/or yeast. This process helps your body better assimilate these foods and increases the amount of beneficial microorganisms in your digestive tract. You need these "good" bacteria for optimal digestion and health, as they also help strengthen your immune system, protect your body from pathogens, and encourage the production of natural antibodies. Fermented foods also help increase the presence of the digestive enzymes that you need to properly digest and absorb nutrients from your food.

Some of the most common fermented foods are tempeh and miso (both made from soy), kimchi and sauerkraut (both made from cabbage), wine, vinegar, yogurt, and kombucha (made from mushrooms).

You'll find recipes for two of my favorite fermented foods—Zesty Kimchi (page 140), and a creamy and delicious Coconut Yogurt (page 131)—in chapter 8.

SWEETENERS

Use these sweeteners and you won't miss white table sugar at all (and you'll certainly never want to eat anything with the dreaded high-fructose corn syrup again!).

Agave

Agave is a thin, mild-tasting syrup derived from certain species of the agave plant. It mixes easily with other ingredients, and as it has a low glycemic index it will not spike your blood sugar. Raw agave contains calcium and small amounts of vitamin C, iron, and magnesium. Be sure, however, to read the labels before you buy, as many brands of agave syrup are not raw, and have been heated to thicken them. See the resources for a list of reputable raw brands.

Brown Rice Syrup

Brown rice syrup is made by fermenting brown rice with added enzymes to release its natural starch properties. The liquid is strained off and then cooked down at very low temperatures until it becomes a sweet syrup. Though it does not retain its fiber, brown rice syrup contains protein and trace minerals. Be sure to read the label to find a pure brown rice syrup that has active enzymes from sprouted barley added into it.

Coconut Nectar and Coconut Crystals

Coconut sweeteners are made from the sap of the coconut palm, just as maple syrup is made from the sap of maple trees. The nectar is liquid, and the crystals resemble sugar. Water from the sap is evaporated without the addition of heat, so the nutrition is retained, including a multitude of amino acids, minerals, B vitamins, vitamin C, essential fatty acids, and enzymes. Both the nectar and the crystals have a neutral pH, which helps keep your body from becoming too acidic. These sweeteners also have low glycemic levels, which will keep your blood sugar on an even keel and prevent the intense blood sugar spikes that make you crave sweets.

Grade B Maple Syrup

Grade B maple syrup is syrup made late in the sugaring season, so it has a higher concentration of nutrients. Not only does it tend to be less expensive than grade A (which is produced in the early part of the season), it is darker, more flavorful, and much higher in minerals. The syrup is a good source of zinc, calcium, manganese, potassium, iron, and magnesium, and offers trace amounts of vitamins B_1, B_2, B_5, and B_6 and folic acid.

Although maple syrup is not a raw sweetener, it is a far more nutritious alternative to commercially processed sugar. Use it in your 20 percent non-raw meals. A little goes a long way!

Raw Honey

Raw honey is an alkaline-forming food and has been shown to regulate blood sugar. It is not heated nor strained, so its natural vitamins, antioxidants, enzymes, and other nutrients are preserved. It has antiviral, antibacterial, and antifungal properties and contains vitamins B_1, B_2, B_3, B_5, B_6, and C. Minerals include magnesium, potassium, calcium, phosphate, sodium chloride, and sulfur. Raw honey boosts energy and is excellent for muscle recovery after rigorous exercise.

Green Leaf Stevia

Stevia is an herb that grows as a shrub in parts of Brazil, Paraguay, China, and Japan. It is about fifteen times sweeter than most sugar but is noncaloric. In addition, it has a long shelf life and is tolerant to high temperatures. It is generally sold in single-serving packets or as a liquid in a dropper bottle. When purchasing green leaf stevia, make sure you are getting the actual natural stevia. Brands like Truvia have been chemically processed.

FATS: THE GOOD KIND

Avocado Oil

Avocado oil is pressed from ripe avocado fruit. It has a rich and buttery taste, and is high in oleic acid, a monounsaturated fatty acid that promotes the body's ability to create antioxidants and has been shown to help improve the cardiovascular system by lowering bad (LDL) cholesterol. Avocado oil provides an abundant amount of vitamin E, is rich in vitamins A, B_1, B_2, and D, and contains omega-6 and omega-3 fatty acids.

Coconut Oil

Extracted from the flesh of ripe coconuts, coconut oil is a saturated fat, but the fat is in the form of medium-chain fatty acids, which are easily converted into energy rather than stored in the body. Coconut oil is extremely hydrating and excellent for the skin and body, both inside and out. As it becomes solid when stored in temperatures below 76°F, it is ideal for skin care uses. Look for cold-pressed coconut oil, which does not use heat in the extraction process.

Extra-Virgin Olive Oil

This is the granddaddy of the healthy oils. Extra-virgin olive oil has antioxidant properties, and has been shown to help reduce inflammation and reduce the risk of heart disease by raising your good (HDL) cholesterol. It is high in monounsaturated fats, including oleic acid, and vitamin E, and contains good amounts of vitamin K, phenols, squalene, and chlorophyll. Cold-pressed olive oils are fun to try because the flavors can vary tremendously depending on the region where the olive oil is produced, just like wine. You can even set up an olive oil tasting at your next dinner party—you'll be amazed at how different the flavors are. Some are fruity; others are peppery, lemony, or earthy.

Flaxseed Oil

Flaxseed oil is made from the seeds of the flax plant. It is an abundant source of omega-3 fatty acids, fiber, and potassium. Studies have shown that flaxseed oil possesses anti-inflammatory properties due to its high concentrate of fatty acids, which help prevent chronic heart disease and arthritis.

Cold-Pressed Sesame Oil

Cold-pressed sesame oil is derived from pressed sesame seeds and is often used in Indian, Korean, or Chinese dishes. It is loaded with omega-6 fatty acids, antioxidants, and antibacterial properties, and has been shown to help regulate the amount of beneficial bacterial in the intestinal tract. It is also high in vitamin K, and is a good source of vitamins E and B_6, magnesium, copper, calcium, iron, and zinc.

CONDIMENTS AND SPICES

There are many ways to spice up your raw kitchen. Try some of these items and your meals will never be boring!

Coconut Aminos

Derived from the sap produced by coconut trees, which is loaded with amino acids and vitamins (C and broad-spectrum B vitamins in particular), this aged liquid bears a close resemblance to soy sauce. It's a good alternative for those watching their salt intake or avoiding soy.

Dulse Flakes

Dulse flakes are made from a red seaweed that has been dried and crushed. Like most seaweeds, dulse is an excellent source of iodine. It's packed with vitamins and minerals such as vitamins A, C, E, and almost all of the B vitamins, calcium, iron, manganese, potassium, and zinc, and it's an excellent source of protein.

Miso

Miso is made by combining soybeans, cultured grains, and sea salt and then double fermenting all the ingredients. It comes in a variety of colors: white, yellow, red, and brown. The darker the color, the saltier and stronger the flavor; white is the mildest, and brown is the strongest. It contains beneficial microorganisms, all the essential amino acids, and probiotics, and is high in antioxidants. It is also high in vitamin B_6, vitamin K, thiamin, riboflavin, iron, magnesium, phosphorus, copper, manganese, and selenium. Most of the recipes in this book use yellow miso, but feel free to try other types depending on your preference. I recommend the brand South River Miso.

Nama Shoyu

If you like soy sauce, you should use only this kind, as it is unpasteurized and contains living enzymes. Though the soybeans are cooked in the brewing process, the product is then fermented, classifying the end product as raw. It is much more flavorful than the soy sauce you might be used to, so a little goes a long way.

Nutritional Yeast

Nutritional yeast has been deactivated, meaning it won't rise like the yeast you use for baking. It is incredibly high in vitamins, including the B-complex vitamins, thiamin, riboflavin, niacin, and folate, and contains iron, magnesium, manganese, and zinc. It is often used by vegans as a cheese substitute, due to its savory taste and smooth, creamy texture when liquid is added.

Sea Salt

Sea salt, quite simply, is the salt that's left behind when seawater is evaporated. Unlike iodized salt, sea salt contains all of the minerals found in seawater, including chloride, sodium, sulfate, magnesium, calcium, and potassium.

Sea Salt—Pink Himalayan

This salt is derived from ancient sea salt deposits and has a higher concentration of minerals than regular sea salt. Its color ranges from white to varying shades of pink and red due to the higher mineral content.

Vinegar—Bragg Organic Apple Cider Vinegar

Made from organic apples, this apple cider vinegar is particularly good for you because it's raw and unfiltered, and contains live enzymes.

Vinegar—Umeboshi

Umeboshi vinegar is a by-product derived from the process of creating Japanese pickled plums. It is fruity, slightly sour, and smells like rich, dark cherries.

ESSENTIAL AND OPTIONAL TOOLS FOR RAW FOOD PREPARATION

Your kitchen cabinets are probably full of pots and pans and lots of utensils for cooking. Well, you'll be able to streamline what you need when you eat a lot of raw food, and you certainly won't have to worry about turning on the stove or oven!

Essential Items

You could go raw with just a good paring knife, if you had to, but that would be a *lot* of work . . . and I want to show you an easier path.

These items are essential for making your food preparation process as speedy and efficient as possible. If you like to cook, you probably already have most if not all of the larger items.

Blender

A blender is an excellent tool for helping to release the beneficial vitamins, nutrients, and enzymes in your food. The more finely chopped food is, the easier it is for your body to absorb. Nearly all blenders will whip up your smoothies in seconds.

Food Processor

A food processor is ideal for cutting up vegetables and making soups, pâtés, and anything with some texture to it. Some have interchangeable blades so you can select how coarse or fine a chop you want, or can grate vegetables quickly. Along with my blender and juicer, my food processor is the most-used item in my kitchen.

Paring and Chef's Knives

The only category where I think it is mandatory to buy the absolute best quality you can afford is knives. A good, sharp knife will last a lifetime, and will be much less likely to cause any harm. You will also chop much more quickly with a sharp, comfortable knife. Find a brand you like, and don't forget to sharpen them often!

Nut-Milk Bags

Nut-milk bags are inexpensive fine mesh bags used for straining and separating the liquid from the pulp of ground nuts. Using them makes the process of making nut milks a breeze.

Vegetable Peeler

A vegetable peeler can quickly slice thin strips from vegetables for use in dishes and salads. Look for one with an ergonomic handle that feels comfortable in your hand.

Optional Items

Dehydrator

A dehydrator uses airflow to remove moisture from food without heating it above 115°F. It is excellent for food preservation, and a great tool to create delicious and satisfying snacks, including crackers, flat breads, chips, fruit leather, veggie burgers, and granola. Learning how to use a dehydrator was what set my business in motion—so I am partial to this marvelous machine! Be careful with the settings, however, as some models allow temperatures as high as 160°F, and you want to stay below 115°F at all times.

Juicer

If you start making and drinking a lot of juice, a juicer is handy to have in your kitchen. It flawlessly removes the pulp (fiber) from fruits and vegetables and allows you to make juice using all the peel and core of fruits (like an apple's), which often are jam-packed with nutrients. If, however, you prefer to drink smoothies with the pulp, you can make do with a blender.

Mandoline

A mandoline is a cutting tool with adjustable and interchangeable blades for slicing fruits and vegetables uniformly in a variety of widths. The blades allow you to quickly julienne, slice, grate, or make crinkle cuts. You can also make longer strips, for use in vegetable "pasta."

Mason Jars

These glass jars with airtight lids are great for storing dry goods in your pantry.

Salad Spinner

A salad spinner removes excess water from leafy greens after you wash them. It usually comes as a plastic tub with an inner basket, and the lid either has a hand crank or cord that you pull. It may seem like a silly device until you use one—and then you realize what a joy it is, especially when you're eating a lot of salads. Removing as much water as possible from your greens keeps them crunchy and extra-delicious.

Spiralizer

Use a spiralizer to uniformly "spiralize" vegetables into long, curly strips perfect for raw pastas or salad garnishes. You can adjust the blade to create strips of varying thicknesses.

8

THE RECIPES

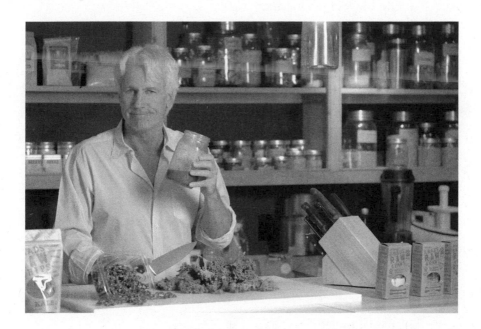

BEVERAGES

SMOOTHIES

Smoothie Basics

- Whenever possible, purchase produce of the highest quality, ideally organic. It's even better if it's local and in season.
- Wash the produce thoroughly with a simple solution of three cups of water to one cup of vinegar. Chop the ingredients into small pieces before blending. Greens such as spinach and kale should be chopped as finely as possible, particularly if your blender isn't very powerful.

- When milk is specified, use rice milk, nut milk, or soy milk. Avoid dairy as much as possible.
- Power up your smoothie with superfoods. See page 105 for suggestions.
- The right blender is the key to creating successful smoothies. Look for a top-rated brand that fits your budget, although you know I love my Vitamix!
- Always add the liquid first because this will make all the ingredients easier to blend. Then you can add smooth solids that blend easily, such as bananas, nut butters, or yogurt. Add chopped-up fruits and/or veggies and seeds last.
- Some recipes call for coconut water. You can use fresh or packaged coconut water. I recommend the Harmless Harvest brand, as it is one of the few raw coconut waters on the market: www .harmlessharvest.com.

SWISS KISS SMOOTHIE

Servings: 2

2 tablespoons lemon juice
1 cup spring water
1 cup raspberries
1 banana, peeled
1 apple, coarsely chopped
3 Swiss chard leaves, stems removed

Place all the ingredients in a blender in the order listed and blend until desired consistency.

ARUGULA AYURVEDA SMOOTHIE

Servings: 2

> 1½ cups coconut water
> 2 pears, coarsely chopped
> 1 handful arugula
> 10 stalks parsley
> 1 (1-inch) piece peeled ginger
> 1 teaspoon ground turmeric powder

Place all the ingredients in a blender in the order listed and blend until desired consistency.

SPINACH SMOOTHIE

Servings: 2

> 2 cups coconut water
> 2 bananas, peeled
> 1 cup blueberries
> 2 cups coarsely chopped pineapple
> 2 cups spinach

Place all the ingredients in a blender in the order listed and blend until desired consistency.

SEÑOR VERDE SMOOTHIE

Servings: 2

> 1 cup orange juice
> ½ avocado, peeled and pitted
> ½ pineapple, peeled, cored, and chopped into chunks
> ½ jalapeño, seeds removed
> 1 handful spinach or 4 kale leaves, ribs removed
> 10 cilantro sprigs
> ½ teaspoon sea salt

Place all the ingredients in a blender in the order listed and blend until desired consistency.

BRAD'S GREEN SMOOTHIE

Servings: 2 meals or 3–4 snacks

3 cups water
2 bananas, peeled
1 pear, coarsely chopped
1 apple, coarsely chopped
1 (1-inch) piece peeled ginger
3 stalks kale, coarsely chopped

Place all the ingredients in a blender in the order listed and blend until desired consistency. Add more water to thin if necessary.

COCO MINT SMOOTHIE

Servings: 2

½ cup coconut water
2 cups nondairy milk
1 avocado, peeled and pitted
¼ cup pitted dates, coarsely chopped
½ vanilla bean, scraped, or 1 teaspoon vanilla extract
¼ cup raw cacao powder
10 fresh mint leaves
1 teaspoon spirulina

Place all the ingredients in a blender in the order listed and blend until desired consistency.

TROPICAL GREEN SMOOTHIE

Servings: 2

2 cups water
1 frozen banana, peeled and chopped into chunks
1 mango, peeled and pitted
2 cups coarsely chopped pineapple
4 handfuls spinach
2 tablespoons hemp seeds (optional)

Place all the ingredients in a blender in the order listed and blend until desired consistency.

BERRY SMOOTHIE

Servings: 2

> 2 cups nondairy milk
> 1 tablespoon lemon juice
> 1 cup strawberries, leaves and stems removed
> 1 cup raspberries
> 1 banana, peeled
> 2 tablespoons sunflower seeds

Place all the ingredients in a blender in the order listed and blend until desired consistency.

CHERRY CACAO SMOOTHIE

Servings: 2

> 2 cups nondairy milk
> 1 teaspoon vanilla extract
> 2 cups pitted sweet cherries
> 2 tablespoons shredded coconut
> ¼ cup cacao nibs

Place all the ingredients in a blender in the order listed and blend until desired consistency.

BANANA CAROB SMOOTHIE

Servings: 2

> 2 cups nondairy milk
> 2 tablespoons coconut oil
> 2 bananas, peeled
> 2 pitted dates, coarsely chopped
> 2 tablespoons carob powder
> ¼ teaspoon Himalayan or regular sea salt

Place all the ingredients in a blender in the order listed and blend until desired consistency.

PEACH PUMP IT UP SMOOTHIE

Servings: 4

> 2 cups nondairy milk
> 2 cups fresh or frozen peach slices
> 1 cup raspberries
> 1 tablespoon maca powder
> 2 tablespoons hemp seeds
> 1 teaspoon nutmeg

Place all the ingredients in a blender in the order listed and blend until desired consistency.

HOW TO MAKE NUT MILK

Fresh nut milk is delicious. Here's how to make it (this makes 3 cups):

- Place 1 cup of nuts or seeds in a bowl and cover with filtered water. Place it in the refrigerator and let it stand overnight.
- Strain and rinse the nuts or seeds and put them in the blender.
- Add 3 cups of filtered water and blend until smooth.
- If you like a sweeter taste, add 2 pitted Medjool dates and blend again. You can add a touch of vanilla as well. Blend again.
- Strain the milk through a nut-milk bag. The pulp will remain in the milk bag. Store the pulp in an airtight container in the refrigerator to use in future smoothies. It's also a great addition to a delicious bowl of fruit!
- Store the nut milk in the refrigerator in an airtight container—a 32-ounce mason jar works well.
- Nut milk will keep in your refrigerator for up to four days, if you can make it last that long. Unlike commercial varieties, it has no emulsifiers or stabilizers, so you'll need to shake it before using.

JUICES

Once produce has been juiced it begins to lose its enzyme content, so consume your juice as quickly as possible in order to reap maximum benefits. If it is more efficient to juice a large quantity at once, a small amount of citrus added to the recipe will help to preserve the nutritional properties for up to seventy-two hours.

When following a juicing recipe, cut the ingredients into pieces that will easily fit into the mouth of the juicer. Start with the greens and stronger flavors (ginger or garlic, for example), adding one ingredient at a time. When using root vegetables such as carrots or beets, scrub them well to remove all dirt, but do not peel the skin before juicing them, as the skin contains a great deal of vitamins and nutrients.

There are many different juicers available, and you can read about some of the options in the resources. But if you do not have a juicer you can still enjoy fresh juices. Throw all the ingredients in your blender and strain the juice with a fine mesh sieve.

BRAD'S GREEN LEMONADE

Servings: 4

4 kale leaves and stalks
1 (½-inch) piece peeled ginger
3 apples, coarsely chopped
1 lemon, peeled
1 cucumber
2 celery stalks

Press the ingredients through the juicer in the order listed.

COLLARD AND PEAR JUICE

Servings: 4

3 collard leaves and stalks
1 (½-inch) piece peeled ginger
2 pears, coarsely chopped
½ lime, peeled
1 cup coconut water

Press the collards, ginger, pears, and lime through the juicer in the order listed. Stir in the coconut water.

GREEN VIBRANCE JUICE

Servings: 2

 2 handfuls spinach
 ½ bunch parsley
 4 celery stalks
 1 cucumber

Press the ingredients through the juicer in the order listed.

MEAN GREEN JUICE

Servings: 2

 6–8 kale leaves and stalks
 1 (1-inch) piece peeled ginger
 4 celery stalks
 ½ lemon, peeled
 1 cucumber
 2 apples

Press the ingredients through the juicer in the order listed.

B8 JUICE

Servings: 2

 4 kale leaves and stalks
 10 parsley sprigs
 ½ lemon, peeled
 2 celery stalks
 1 beet, quartered
 6 carrots
 1 zucchini
 3 oranges, peeled

Press the ingredients through the juicer in the order listed.

CUCUMBER JUICE

Servings: 1

6 kale leaves and stalks
1 cucumber
Small bundle parsley
Small bundle mint
2 limes, peeled
1 cucumber

Press the ingredients through the juicer in the order listed.

KALE WITH A KICK! JUICE

Servings: 2

6 celery stalks with leaves
4 kale leaves and stalks
1 handful cilantro or parsley with stems
2 (1-inch) pieces peeled ginger
1 lemon, peeled
1 cucumber
4 Granny Smith apples

Press the ingredients through the juicer in the order listed.

BRAD'S WAKE-UP JUICE

Servings: 2

4 kale leaves and stalks
1 (½-inch) piece peeled ginger
2–3 celery stalks
1 lime, peeled
1 large cucumber
Pinch cayenne pepper

Press the kale, ginger, celery, lime, and cucumber through the juicer. Add the cayenne and stir thoroughly.

BLOODY MARY JUICE

Servings: 2

>   10 parsley sprigs
>   1 (½-inch) piece peeled ginger or fresh horseradish
>   2 celery stalks
>   2 small tomatoes
>   ¼ cup lemon juice

Press the parsley, ginger, celery, and tomatoes through the juicer. Add the lemon juice and stir to combine. (If you'd rather use horseradish instead of ginger and fresh horseradish is not available, use jarred, finely minced horseradish, and stir it into the juice at the end.)

VITALITY JUICE

Servings: 2

>   3 kale leaves and stalks
>   1 (1-inch) piece peeled ginger
>   2 garlic cloves
>   ½ fennel bulb
>   3 celery stalks
>   1 carrot
>   1 bunch sprouts, your choice
>   ½ cucumber
>   Pinch cayenne pepper

Press the kale, ginger, garlic, fennel, celery, carrot, sprouts, and cucumber through the juicer. Add the cayenne and stir thoroughly.

APPLE PIE JUICE

Servings: 2

>   4 carrots
>   6 apples
>   ¼ teaspoon nutmeg

Press the carrots and apples through the juicer. Stir in the nutmeg.

GRAPE-ADE JUICE
Servings: 2

1 bunch celery, ends trimmed
1 lemon, peeled
1 lime, peeled
2½ cups grapes
2 apples, coarsely chopped

Press the ingredients through the juicer in the order listed.

BRAD'S REHYDRATION JUICE
Servings: 2

6 celery stalks
1 lime, peeled
⅔ cup chopped pineapple
1 green apple, coarsely chopped

Press the ingredients through the juicer in the order listed.

WATERMELON, PINEAPPLE, AND GINGER JUICE
Servings: 2

⅓ pineapple, peeled, cored, and chopped into chunks
1 (1-inch) piece peeled ginger
2 large watermelon slices, seeds and rind removed

Press the ingredients through the juicer in the order listed.

PINEAPPLE BASIL MOCKTAIL
Servings: 4

1 pineapple, peeled, cored, and chopped into chunks
1 small handful basil leaves
1 cup sparkling water

Place the pineapple and basil in a blender; blend until smooth. Strain the mixture into a pitcher, add the sparkling water, and stir gently to combine. Serve immediately.

CHAMPAGNE

Servings: 4

> 4 cups white grape juice
> 2 cups pineapple juice
> ¼ cup lemon juice
> ¼ cup lime juice
> 3–4 tablespoons agave nectar
> 6 cups sparkling water

In a large pitcher stir together the grape, pineapple, lemon, and lime juices. Stir in the agave. Fill 4 champagne glasses ⅓ full with the juice mixture and fill each glass to the brim with sparkling water.

MOCKARITA

Servings: 4

> 1 teaspoon lime juice
> Juice of 1 orange
> 1 cup pineapple juice
> 1 teaspoon agave nectar
> ¾ cup sparkling water

Fill a cocktail shaker ¾ of the way full with crushed ice. Pour in the lime juice, then add the orange juice, pineapple juice, agave, and sparkling water. Shake the shaker and pour drinks into margarita glasses.

BREAKFAST

COCONUT YOGURT

Note: This recipe can be made only with a dehydrator.

Makes 1 quart

>   4 cups canned coconut milk (light or whole)
>   1 packet or 0.125 grams of yogurt culture*

Pour the coconut milk into a glass bowl and whisk in the yogurt culture. Put the bowl in the dehydrator and set the dehydrator at 95°F for 6–12 hours (the longer it sits, the tangier the taste). Remove and store in an airtight container in the refrigerator for up to 2 weeks.

*My favorite vegan yogurt culture is from Cultures for Health. Other vegetarian cultures are Wilderness Family Naturals and Body Ecology.

MATURE COCONUT MILK (WHOLE FAT)

Makes 1 quart

>   2 mature coconuts
>   4 cups fresh coconut water

Pierce the soft eyes of the coconuts, drain the liquid into a container, and reserve. Wrap each coconut in a kitchen towel, place it on a solid countertop or on the floor, and strike it with a hammer until the shell cracks in two. Using a butter knife or oyster knife, scrape the meat out and place it in a blender. Pour in the coconut water and blend on high for at least 2 minutes. This will warm the milk slightly, which will make it easier to strain. Strain it through a nut-milk bag and discard the solids. Store the milk in an airtight container in the refrigerator for up to 2 weeks.

FRESH SPROUTED BREAKFAST CEREAL

Servings: 4

> 2 cups buckwheat, sprouted for 1 day only
> 1 cup sunflower seeds, sprouted for 1 day only
> ½ cup of your favorite dried fruit, chopped small
> ¼ cup cacao nibs
> ½ teaspoon lemon juice
> 1 teaspoon vanilla extract
> 2 tablespoons maple syrup

Mix all the ingredients together and keep in an airtight container in the refrigerator for up to 2 weeks. Or for a crunchy cereal, dehydrate at 110°F for 6–12 hours. Add to a bowl with nut milk and enjoy.

ENERGY BARS

Servings: 6

> 1 pound pitted dates
> ½ cup sprouted sunflower seeds
> ½ cup sprouted almonds
> 1 (1-inch) piece peeled ginger
> ½ cup hemp seeds
> 4 tablespoons maca powder
> ½ cup cacao powder
> 1 teaspoon sea salt
> 1 cup unsweetened coconut flakes
> 4 tablespoons coconut oil
> 2 tablespoons raw honey
> 1 mashed banana

Put all the ingredients into a food processor and pulse until coarsely ground. Press the mixture into an 8 x 8-inch pan and place it in the refrigerator for at least 4 hours. Cut it into 6 bars before serving.

BRAD'S BREAKFAST QUINOA

Servings: 4

1 cup quinoa
Almond milk
1 tablespoon slivered almonds
1 tablespoon dried berries
1 teaspoon hemp seeds
1 teaspoon cinnamon
1 teaspoon nutmeg

Cook the quinoa following package directions. Scoop out ½ cup cooked quinoa into a small pan and add a few splashes of almond milk. (The remainder can be stored in the refrigerator in an airtight container for 4 days.) Reheat over low heat on the stove. Top with almonds, berries, and hemp seeds. Sprinkle with cinnamon and nutmeg.

Variation: For a raw version, place ½ cup sprouted quinoa in a bowl and add almond milk to taste.

MORNING CORN SOUP

Servings: 2

2 cups fresh corn kernels
1 cup coconut milk (whole or low fat)
1 teaspoon yellow miso paste
½ avocado, peeled, pitted, and coarsely chopped
1 tablespoon coconut oil, melted
Juice of ½ lime
1 small jalapeño, seeded and deveined, finely chopped
1½ teaspoons sea salt
Freshly ground black pepper, to taste

Place the ingredients in a food processor and pulse a few times until the consistency is similar to gazpacho; the soup is best when the texture is slightly chunky.

APPETIZERS, SNACKS, AND SIDES

RAWCHO CHEESE

Makes 2 cups

> 1 cup cashews, soaked overnight and drained
> ¼ red bell pepper, coarsely chopped
> 3 tablespoons olive oil
> 2 tablespoons yellow miso
> 2 tablespoons lemon juice
> ½ teaspoon sea salt
> 1 teaspoon minced white onion
> ¼ teaspoon turmeric
> 1 tablespoon raw hot sauce (optional)

Place all the ingredients in a blender and blend at high speed until smooth. Store in an airtight container in the refrigerator for up to 4 days.

CHIVE-MISO FLAX CRACKERS

Note: This recipe can be made only with a dehydrator.

Servings: 4

> 2 cups whole flaxseeds, soaked for 2–6 hours and drained
> ¼ cup nama shoyu
> 2 tablespoons yellow miso
> ½ cup minced chives
> 1 tablespoon lime juice

Place the flaxseeds in a bowl and stir in the nama shoyu, miso, chives, and lime juice. Spread the mixture about 1/8 inch thick on the dehydrator trays and dehydrate at 110°F for 4–6 hours. Turn the mixture over, and dehydrate another 3–4 hours. If you like a crispy and crunchy cracker, dehydrate a bit longer. I like my flaxseed crackers a bit chewier, so I dehydrate them a bit less. Break or slice your crackers into pieces when they are finished dehydrating.

PINE NUT CHEESE

Makes 1½ cups

> 1 cup pine nuts, soaked overnight and drained
>
> 3 tablespoons nutritional yeast flakes
>
> ½ teaspoon sea salt
>
> ½ teaspoon lemon zest
>
> 1 tablespoon lemon juice

Place all the ingredients in a food processor and blend until smooth. Store in an airtight container in the refrigerator for up to 4 days.

ZESTY FLAX CRACKERS

Note: This recipe can be made only with a dehydrator.

Servings: 4

> 8 cups golden flaxseeds, soaked for 6 hours and drained
>
> 4–5 carrots, scrubbed and rinsed
>
> 6–7 celery stalks, leaves and ribs removed
>
> 1½ red bell peppers, stemmed and seeded
>
> ½ large onion
>
> 1 bunch cilantro, stems removed
>
> 1 large tomato, cored and coarsely chopped
>
> Sea salt, to taste
>
> 3 teaspoons cumin
>
> 2 teaspoons cayenne pepper or chipotle powder

Place the flaxseeds, carrots, celery, red peppers, onion, and cilantro in a food processor and pulse until combined. Add the tomato and pulse once or twice. Add the sea salt, cumin, and cayenne and pulse to combine. Spread the mixture about 1/8 inch thick on the dehydrator trays and dehydrate at 110°F for 4–6 hours. Turn the mixture over, and dehydrate another 3–4 hours. If you like a crispy and crunchy cracker, dehydrate a bit longer. I like my flaxseed crackers a bit chewier, so I dehydrate them a bit less. Break or slice your crackers into pieces when they are finished dehydrating. Store any extra batter in the fridge (up to a week) for future use.

CRAIC NUTS

Note: This recipe can be made only with a dehydrator.

Makes 2 cups

> 2 cups pecans, soaked overnight, drained, and rinsed well
> ⅓ cup maple syrup
> 1 tablespoon coconut oil
> 1 tablespoon garam masala spice blend
> ½ teaspoon sea salt

Dry the pecans in a dehydrator at 110°F for 4 hours. Place dried nuts in a bowl and mix with maple syrup, oil, spice, and salt. Dehydrate at 110°F for another 8 hours or until crisp.

SEA KALE CHIPS

Note: This recipe can be made only with a dehydrator.

Servings: 4

> 1 bunch kale, washed and dried
> 1 tablespoon lemon juice
> Pinch cayenne pepper
> 1 tablespoon dulse flakes
> 2 tablespoons olive oil

Remove the kale leaves from the stalks, leaving the greens in large pieces, and place the greens in a large mixing bowl. In a small bowl, whisk the lemon juice, cayenne, dulse, and olive oil together and pour the mixture over the kale. Massage kale with the dressing. Dehydrate at 115°F for 4 hours or until crisp.

EGGPLANT BACON

Note: This recipe can be made only with a dehydrator.

Servings: 4

  1 chipotle pepper, stem removed
  1 tablespoon smoked paprika
  1 teaspoon freshly ground black pepper
  1 tablespoon maple syrup
  2 tablespoons extra-virgin olive oil
  1 tablespoon coconut oil
  3 tablespoons nama shoyu
  1 large eggplant, peeled and sliced paper thin on a mandoline

Place the chipotle, paprika, black pepper, maple syrup, olive oil, co-conut oil, and nama shoyu in a blender and blend until emulsified. Place the eggplant slices in a bowl and toss with the blended marinade until well coated. Let marinate for 30 minutes. Layer evenly on trays to dehydrate at 115°F for 12 hours, then remove the teflex sheet, and continue drying for several more hours until the eggplant is crisp.

FOCACCIA

Note: This recipe can be made only with a dehydrator.

Servings: 4

  2 carrots, peeled and chopped coarsely
  1 medium zucchini, chopped coarsely
  1 cup sunflower seeds, soaked overnight and drained
  1 yellow onion, chopped coarsely
  1 cup coarsely chopped sun-dried tomatoes
  ½ cup ground flaxseed
  ½ cup extra-virgin olive oil
  2 tablespoons yellow miso
  3 tablespoons nama shoyu
  2 tablespoons Italian seasoning or a blend of oregano, thyme, basil,
     and rosemary

Place all the ingredients in a food processor and blend until smooth. Spread the mixture about 1 inch thick on the dehydrator tray and dehydrate at 105°F for 18–24 hours. Cut into desired sizes for sandwiches or snacks.

GREEN SEEDS

Note: This recipe can be made only with a dehydrator.

Makes 2 cups

2 cups sprouted sunflower seeds, soaked overnight and drained
1 tablespoon spirulina
1 teaspoon turmeric
½ teaspoon cayenne pepper
¼ teaspoon freshly ground black pepper
½ teaspoon sea salt

Spread sprouted seeds on a dehydrator tray. Dehydrate overnight at 115°F. In a bowl, mix dried seeds with spirulina, turmeric, cayenne, black pepper, and salt. Let sit for at least 4 hours. Place the mixture back on a dehydrator tray and dehydrate again for 12 hours at 100°F. Store in an airtight container. Use as a snack or a salad topper.

ONION BREAD

Note: This recipe can be made only with a dehydrator.

Servings: 4

3 cups chia seeds, soaked in 6 cups of water for 1 hour and drained
5 onions, 3 minced in a food processor and 2 thinly sliced
1 cup pitted raw Greek olives, pureed in a food processor
½ cup parsley leaves, minced

Place the chia seeds in a bowl and fold in the minced onions and pureed olives. Spread the mixture about ½ inch thick on the dehydrator tray. Evenly layer slices of onions on the mixture and sprinkle parsley on top. Dehydrate at 110°F for 6 hours, then remove the bread from the trays, cut it into 2-inch squares, and continue dehydrating for another day or until desired firmness is reached.

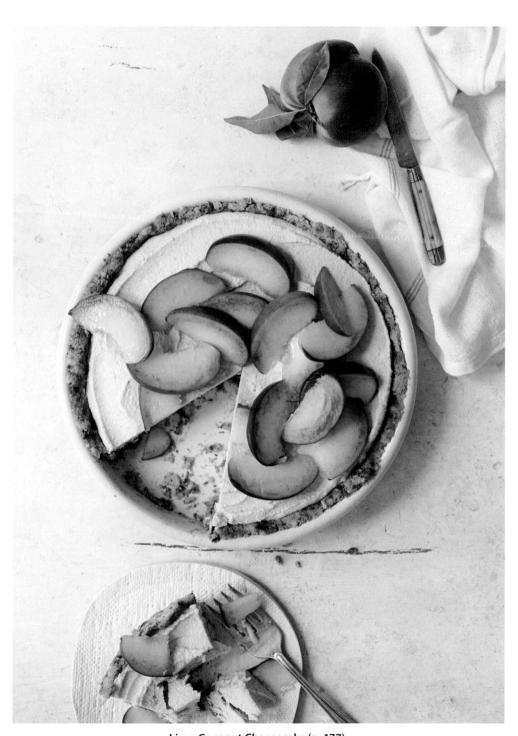

Lime Coconut Cheesecake (p. 177)

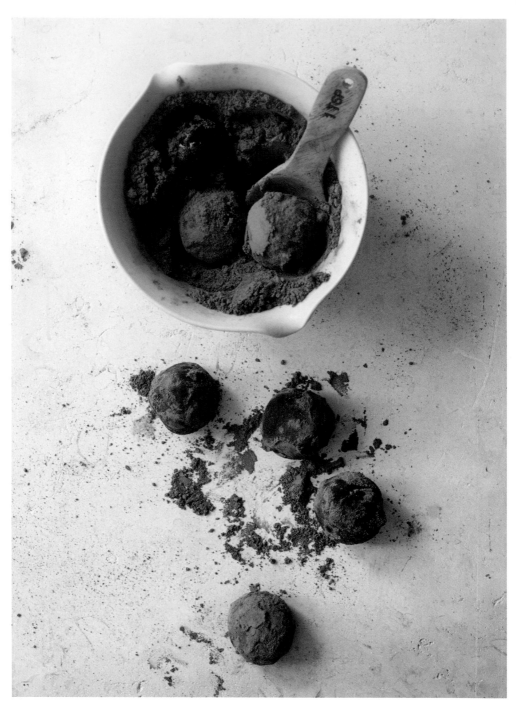

Mayan Chocolate Truffles (p. 180)

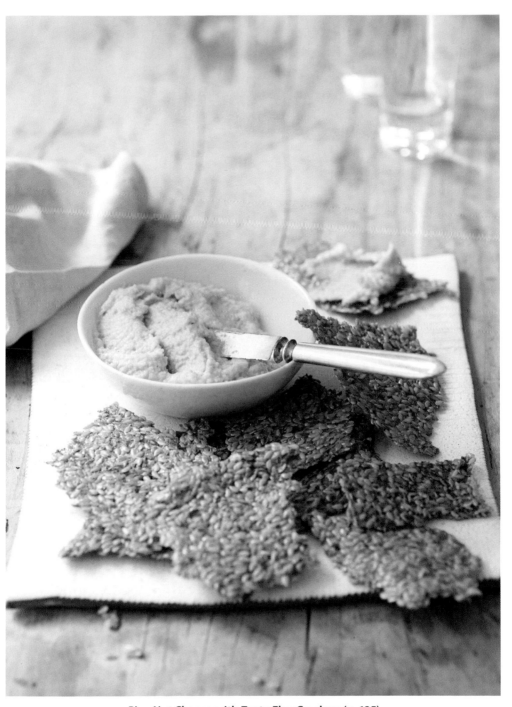

Pine Nut Cheese with Zesty Flax Crackers (p. 135)

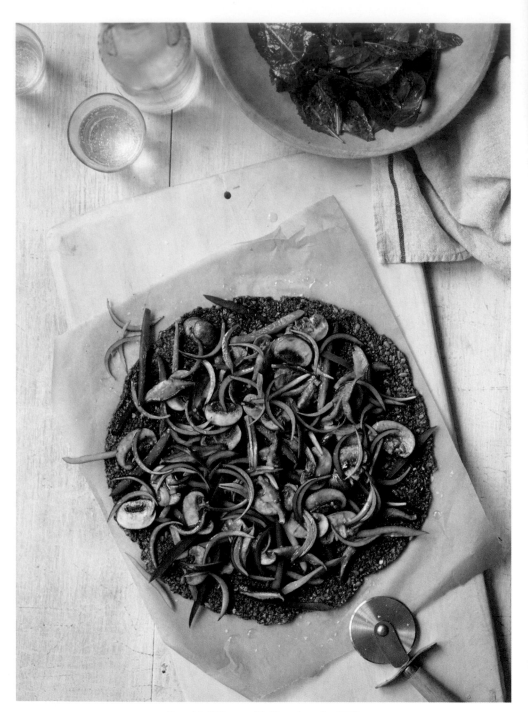

Zucchini Pizza with Toppings (p. 168)

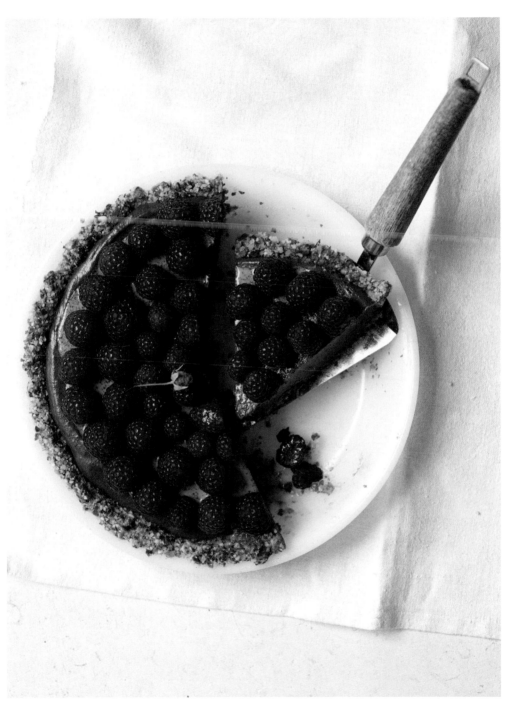

Chocolate Mousse Pie (p. 182)

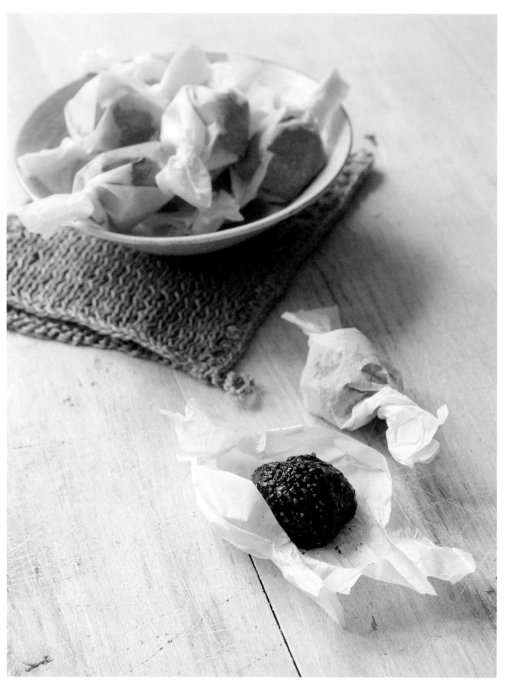

Miah's Energy Balls (p. 170)

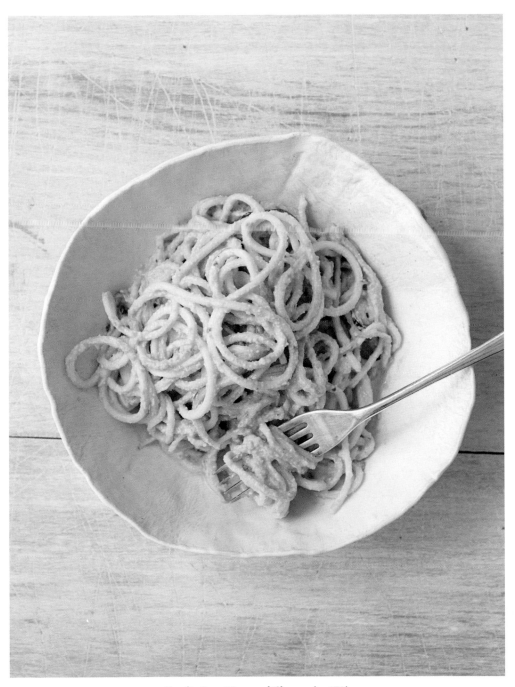

Brad's Raw Mac and Cheese (p. 173)

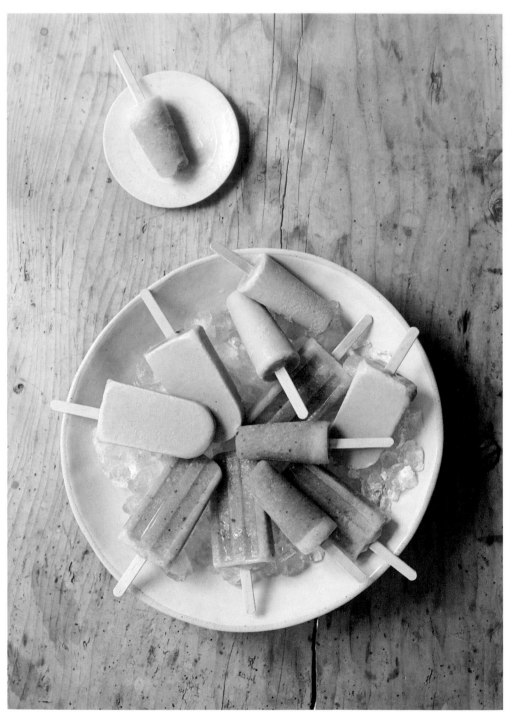

Brad's Frozen Green Smoothie Pops (p. 173) and Brazil Nut Mylk Gone Wild! pops (p. 172)

JICAMA FRIES

Servings: 4

1 jicama, peeled and sliced into ½-inch strips
1 tablespoon olive oil
1 tablespoon paprika
½ teaspoon sea salt
1 teaspoon lemon zest
Juice of 1 lemon

Place the jicama in a bowl. Add the oil, paprika, salt, lemon zest, and lemon juice and toss well to coat. The fries can be dehydrated at 115°F for 12 hours for a crispier texture. They are perfect when paired with Raw Ketchup (page 145).

CORN SUCCOTASH

Servings: 4

SUCCOTASH
2 cups corn kernels
1 cup sprouted sunflower seeds
¼ cup chopped cilantro
½ cup diced celery
½ cup diced zucchini
½ cup diced tomato
½ cup finely chopped red onion

DRESSING
¼ cup extra-virgin olive oil
1 tablespoon raw honey
¼ teaspoon stone-ground mustard
1 teaspoon sea salt
Freshly ground black pepper, to taste

In a bowl combine the corn, sunflower seeds, cilantro, celery, zucchini, tomato, and onion and set aside. For the dressing, pour the olive oil and honey into a small jar, and add the mustard, salt, and pepper. Cover and shake together until the dressing is emulsified. Pour it over the succotash and toss well.

ZESTY KIMCHI

Makes 2 quarts

⅓ cup plus 1 tablespoon sea salt

1 large head napa or green cabbage, cored and chopped coarsely

1 carrot, peeled and chopped coarsely

3 garlic cloves

1 (1-inch) piece peeled ginger

10 cilantro leaves and stems

4 scallions, ends and dark green parts trimmed, chopped coarsely

1 teaspoon cayenne pepper

1 teaspoon lime zest

¼ cup water

Fill a large mixing bowl full of water, add ⅓ cup sea salt, and stir to dissolve. Soak cabbage in salt water for 30 minutes then drain in a colander. Place the carrot, garlic, ginger, cilantro, and scallions in a food processor and pulse until coarsely shredded. Put the mixture into a large bowl and add the cayenne, lime zest, remaining sea salt, and water. Add the cabbage and mix well. Transfer the mixture to a half-gallon mason jar. Press the mixture down until liquid rises to the top. Screw the lid on tightly and let it sit and ferment for at least 4 days—longer for more flavor. A little white mold may appear; this is harmless and can be mixed in. When stored in an airtight container in the refrigerator, kimchi can last for several months. If the cabbage becomes soggy and starts to taste too strongly fermented, or becomes too fizzy, it's time to discard.

HUMMUS FRESCO

Servings: 6

2 zucchini, peeled and coarsely chopped

¾ cup raw tahini

½ cup pine nuts, soaked overnight and drained

⅓ cup fresh lemon juice

¼ cup extra-virgin olive oil

4 garlic cloves, peeled

2 teaspoons sea salt

1 tablespoon ground cumin

Place all ingredients in a food processor and blend until smooth.

BRAD'S KICKIN' GUACAMOLE

Servings: 2

1 avocado
1 small tomato, cored and chopped
1 tablespoon minced white onion
4 tablespoons minced cilantro
2 tablespoons lime juice
1 jalapeño, seeded and chopped
1 teaspoon sea salt

Scoop the avocado flesh into a bowl and break it up into chunks with a fork. Add the tomato, onion, cilantro, lime juice, jalapeño, and salt. Using a wooden spoon, mix the ingredients together. You want a chunky consistency.

How to Make Pickled Red Cabbage

1 head red cabbage
2 tablespoons salt
10 cups white vinegar
6 tablespoons pickling spice

Cut the cabbage in half lengthwise, then into quarters. Slice it into very thin slices. Toss the cabbage in a large bowl with the salt. Place a plate on top of the cabbage and top it with a heavy weight to pack it down. After 24 hours, place the vinegar and pickling spices in a pot and bring to a boil. Boil for 6 minutes. Remove the plate from the top of the cabbage and pack the cabbage into glass canning jars, leaving an inch of room at the top. Pour the hot liquid over the cabbage so that it's covered. Place lids on the jars and close tightly. Store in the refrigerator for 6 days. It will then be ready to eat.

Note: The jars do not need to be sterilized, as this is not typical canning or pickling.

SUPERFOOD APRICOT BAR

Servings: 6

> 1 cup macadamia nuts, soaked overnight and drained
> 1 cup pistachio nuts, soaked overnight and drained
> ½ cup sunflower seeds, soaked overnight and drained
> 1½ cups finely chopped dried apricots
> ½ cup finely chopped pitted dates
> ½ cup goji berries
> Pinch sea salt
> 1½ cups dried unsweetened shredded coconut
> 2 tablespoons vanilla extract
> 2 tablespoons coconut milk

Combine the macadamia nuts, pistachios, and sunflower seeds in a food processor and pulse until finely ground. Then add the chopped apricots, dates, goji berries, and salt; pulse and process all the ingredients together until coarsely ground. Add the shredded coconut and give a quick pulse. Add the vanilla and milk until all the ingredients are incorporated. Place the dough mixture into a pan lined with parchment paper, press it in an even layer, and chill for at least 2 hours before serving. Cut the mixture into bars and individually wrap them for snacks on the go.

CAULIFLOWER POPCORN

Servings: 4

> 1 whole cauliflower, cored and chopped in popcorn-size pieces
> 4–8 tablespoons nutritional yeast
> Sea salt and freshly ground black pepper, to taste
> 2 tablespoons extra-virgin olive oil
> 1 tablespoon coconut oil, melted
> 1 tablespoon spirulina
> ¼ teaspoon cayenne pepper

Place all the ingredients in a gallon-size zip-top bag. Now shake the bag until your arms hurt. You can make the popcorn cheesier by adding more yeast, greener by adding more spirulina.

You can eat the Cauliflower Popcorn as is, which I usually do, or you can dehydrate it for 6–8 hours at 115°F, and it will shrink up into yummy little crunchy pieces. Be sure to go easy on the salt if you dehydrate it, as the flavors will intensify.

PÂTÉ ROSA

Servings: 6

2 cups walnuts, soaked overnight and drained
½ medium tomato
1 sun-dried tomato
½ red bell pepper, stemmed and seeded
2 tablespoons lemon juice
1 tablespoon cumin
2 pinches of salt

Place all the ingredients in a food processor and blend until everything is mixed well. Pour into a lightly oiled 5 x 8-inch loaf pan and chill overnight. To serve, run a knife along the edge of the pan to loosen the pâté, then invert the loaf pan onto a flat dish, giving it a few quick shakes side to side so that the pâté comes out in one piece. Slice the pâté and serve on veggies, sprouted bread, or crackers.

ZA'ATAR ALMOND OLIVE PÂTÉ

Servings: 4

2 cups almond pulp, left over from making nut milk (page 124)
⅓ cup extra-virgin olive oil, plus additional for finishing
½ cup kalamata olives, pitted
¼ cup lemon juice
2 garlic cloves
½ cup diced red bell pepper
1 tablespoon za'atar spice blend, plus additional for finishing

Place all the ingredients in a food processor and process until smooth. Scoop out the mixture into a bowl, drizzle with olive oil, add a sprinkle of more za'atar spice, and serve with bread or crackers.

CONDIMENTS, DRESSINGS, AND SAUCES

CONDIMENTS

SPIRULINA SEAWEED GOMASIO

Makes 1 cup

1 tablespoon spirulina
½ cup hemp seeds
½ cup sesame seeds
1 teaspoon sea salt
2 tablespoons dulse flakes

Combine all the ingredients in a small bowl. Pour the mixture into a shaker and use as seasoning.

RAW MAYONNAISE

Makes 2 cups

1 cup cashews, soaked for 1–6 hours and drained
¼ cup water
4 tablespoons freshly squeezed lemon juice
6 tablespoons raw vinegar
1 tablespoon raw honey
2 teaspoons minced white onion
2 teaspoons salt
Pinch freshly ground black pepper
1 teaspoon raw mustard
3 tablespoons extra-virgin olive oil
3 tablespoons flaxseed oil

Combine the cashews, water, lemon juice, vinegar, honey, onion, salt, pepper, and mustard in a blender and process until smooth. With the blender running, add the oils in a steady stream until they are emulsified. If the mixture is too thick, add more water a teaspoon at a time until the mayonnaise is thinner. Stored in the refrigerator, this will keep for up to 4 weeks.

BBQ SAUCE

Makes 3 cups

1 cup sun-dried tomatoes, soaked for 1–2 hours and drained

5 tablespoons apple cider vinegar

½ teaspoon smoked paprika

½ teaspoon finely ground sea salt

1 tablespoon flaxseed oil

2 garlic cloves

2 tablespoons finely chopped white onion

2 tablespoons nama shoyu

2 tablespoons lemon juice

12 pitted dates, soaked in 1 cup of coconut water for 1–2 hours, undrained

Pinch cayenne pepper

1 tablespoon mesquite powder (optional)

Place all the ingredients in a food processor and pulse until smooth. Store in an airtight container in the refrigerator for up to 1 week.

RAW KETCHUP

Makes 2 cups

1½ cups chopped tomatoes

3 tablespoons coarsely chopped, pitted dates

¼ cup extra-virgin olive oil

2 tablespoons dulse flakes

1 tablespoon chopped white onion

1 garlic clove

¼ teaspoon ground cloves

1 teaspoon sea salt

1 tablespoon apple cider vinegar

½ cup sun-dried tomatoes

Place all the ingredients in a blender and blend until smooth. Store in the refrigerator for up to 1 week.

BRAD'S ZINGIN' HOT SAUCE

Makes 1½ cups

2 tablespoons ground dried chipotle chiles
3 fresh jalapeño peppers, seeded
1 carrot, peeled and chopped coarsely
1 tablespoon freshly ground black pepper
½ cup filtered water
2 tablespoons apple cider vinegar
1 tablespoon sea salt

Place all the ingredients in a blender and puree until smooth.

Variation: To make this a tropical hot sauce, add ½ cup chopped mango to the ingredients.

SALAD DRESSINGS

BRAD'S HOUSE DRESSING

Makes 3½ cups

¼ cup sunflower seeds, soaked overnight and drained
½ cup cashews
1–2 jalapeños, seeded and chopped
2 carrots, peeled and shredded
2 red bell peppers, seeded and cored
2 tablespoons lemon juice
½ zucchini, ends trimmed, chopped
2 tablespoons nama shoyu
1 teaspoon Himalayan or regular sea salt
1 handful cilantro
2 tablespoons lemon juice
Water to thin
Black pepper, to taste

Place all the ingredients in a blender and puree on high for about 30 seconds until completely smooth.

SUN-DRIED TOMATO AND KALAMATA DRESSING

Makes 2 cups

> ½ can sun-dried tomatoes, rehydrated (soak in lukewarm water for
>   one hour) and drained
> 1 cup extra-virgin olive oil
> ¼ cup vinegar
> ½ handful fresh basil leaves
> ¾ cup raw kalamata olives, pitted and coarsely chopped
> 2 garlic cloves
> Pinch cayenne pepper (optional)

Place all the ingredients in a blender and process until desired consistency.

BABY BASIL DRESSING

Makes 1½ cups

> 1 tablespoon fresh, chopped basil
> ½ teaspoon tamari
> ½ cup apple cider vinegar
> ½ tablespoon fresh oregano
> 1 tablespoon lemon juice
> 1 cup extra-virgin olive oil

Place the basil, tamari, vinegar, oregano, and lemon juice in a blender. Start the blender on low speed, and drizzle in the olive oil ¼ cup at a time while blending.

THAI DREAM DRESSING

Makes 1½ cups

> ¼ cup sesame oil
> ½ cup nama shoyu or coconut aminos
> ¼ cup extra-virgin olive oil
> ¼ cup lime juice
> 2 tablespoons raw vinegar
> 1 tablespoon coconut crystals or raw honey
> ½ jalapeño, seeded

2 tablespoons dulse flakes

1 small handful cilantro leaves

1 small handful fresh basil leaves

¼ cup cashews, soaked for 2–6 hours and drained

Place all the ingredients in a blender and process for 30 seconds or until you get a creamy consistency.

MISO HAPPY DRESSING

Makes 1½ cups

⅓ cup coarsely chopped Vidalia onion

1 small garlic clove, chopped

1 carrot, peeled and coarsely chopped

⅓ cup yellow miso

¼ cup raw tahini

3 tablespoons nama shoyu or coconut aminos

1 tablespoon lemon juice

2 tablespoons vinegar

2 tablespoons raw honey

½ cup coconut water

1 (½-inch) piece peeled ginger

Place all the ingredients in a blender and process for about 30 seconds or until smooth.

CAESAR DRESSING

Makes 1½ cups

¼ cup sunflower seeds, soaked overnight and drained

⅛ cup pine nuts, soaked overnight and drained

3 tablespoons lemon juice

¼ cup cold-pressed extra-virgin olive oil

3 garlic cloves

1 heaping tablespoon yellow miso

½ teaspoon sea salt

½ teaspoon kelp granules

½ teaspoon dulse flakes

Freshly ground black pepper, to taste

¼ cup water

Place all the ingredients in a blender and process until it reaches the desired consistency.

GRAPEFRUIT STAR DRESSING

Makes 1½ cups

> Juice of 1 large grapefruit
> Juice of 1 navel orange
> ½ cup extra-virgin olive oil
> ¼ cup flaxseed oil
> 2 tablespoons raw honey
> 1 tablespoon raw vinegar
> 1 teaspoon sea salt
> 1 (1-inch) piece peeled ginger
> ½ teaspoon ground star anise

Place all the ingredients in a blender and process until it reaches the desired consistency.

CREAMY GREEN DRESSING

Makes 1½ cups

> 2 tablespoons dulse flakes
> 1 garlic clove, peeled and chopped
> ¼ avocado, peeled and pitted
> 1 cup coconut water
> ½ cup loosely packed fresh Italian parsley leaves
> ¼ cup loosely packed fresh tarragon leaves
> 2 tablespoons finely chopped fresh chives
> 3 tablespoons lemon juice
> 3 tablespoons nama shoyu
> Freshly ground black pepper, to taste

Place all the ingredients in a blender and process until it reaches the desired consistency.

GREEK HERB LEMON DRESSING

Makes 1½ cups

½ cup extra-virgin olive oil

1 tablespoon red wine vinegar

1 teaspoon lemon zest

½ cucumber, peeled and seeded

1 tablespoon lemon juice

2 tablespoons finely chopped fresh oregano or marjoram leaves

1 small handful parsley leaves

1 garlic clove, chopped

¼ red onion, coarsely chopped

1 teaspoon stone-ground mustard

½ teaspoon sea salt

Place all the ingredients in a blender and blend for about 30 seconds or until it reaches the desired consistency.

HONEY MUSTARD DRESSING

Makes 1½ cups

2 tablespoons stone-ground mustard

2 tablespoons raw honey

1 cup Raw Mayonnaise (page 144)

1 teaspoon lime juice

¼ teaspoon turmeric

Pinch cayenne pepper

Place all the ingredients in a bowl and whisk until smooth.

FENNEL VINAIGRETTE

Makes 1 cup

1 cup chopped fennel

2 teaspoons chopped fennel fronds

5 tablespoons raw vinegar

1 tablespoon parsley leaves

2 tablespoons chopped shallots

1 teaspoon sea salt

¼ teaspoon freshly ground black pepper
¼ cup water
½ cup extra-virgin olive oil

Place all the ingredients in a blender and process until desired consistency is reached.

RAITA

Makes 2 cups

2 cups Coconut Yogurt (page 131)
3 tablespoons chopped fresh mint
1 teaspoon cumin
¼ teaspoon chili powder
1 tablespoon nama shoyu
¼ teaspoon cayenne pepper
½ teaspoon lemon juice

Place all the ingredients in a blender and puree until smooth.

SAUCES

All sauces should be refrigerated in airtight containers when not in use, and should be consumed within 4–5 days.

PUTTANESCA SAUCE

Makes 2½ cups

¼ cup sun-dried tomatoes, soaked overnight and drained
2 cups coarsely chopped fresh tomatoes, divided use
Pinch sea salt (optional)
¼ cup olive oil–cured olives
2 tablespoons salted capers, soaked overnight and drained
2 garlic cloves, chopped
2 tablespoons olive oil
¼ cup finely chopped flat-leaf parsley
Freshly ground black pepper, to taste

Place the sun-dried tomatoes, 1 cup of the fresh tomatoes, and sea salt in a blender and blend until smooth. Pour the mixture into a bowl and add the remaining fresh tomatoes, olives, capers, garlic, olive oil, parsley, and black pepper. Great over Veggie Ribbon Noodles (page 166).

MACADAMIA ALFREDO SAUCE

Makes 3 cups

    1 cup macadamia nuts, soaked overnight and drained
    1 teaspoon raw honey
    3 tablespoons lemon juice
    ½ teaspoon sea salt
    2 tablespoons finely chopped parsley leaves
    ½ teaspoon freshly ground black pepper
    1 garlic clove, chopped
    1¼ cups nut milk
    ¼ cup nutritional yeast

Place all the ingredients in a blender and process until the desired consistency is reached.

PESTO

Makes 1 cup

    ¾ cup walnuts, soaked overnight and drained
    2 packed cups fresh basil leaves
    6 tablespoons extra-virgin olive oil
    1 tablespoon lemon juice
    2 garlic cloves, chopped
    1 teaspoon sea salt

Place all the ingredients in a blender and process until the desired consistency is reached.

MARINARA SAUCE

Makes 4 cups

2 tablespoons olive oil

5 fresh tomatoes, cored

½ cup sun-dried tomatoes, soaked overnight and drained

3 garlic cloves, chopped

2 tablespoons finely chopped onion

½ cup finely chopped fresh basil leaves

1 tablespoon fresh oregano or marjoram

½ teaspoon sea salt, plus additional to taste

Freshly ground black pepper, to taste

Place the olive oil, fresh tomatoes, sun-dried tomatoes, garlic, onion, basil, oregano, and salt in a blender and process until the desired consistency is reached. Add additional salt and pepper to taste.

SALADS

FENNEL AND ORANGE SALAD

Servings: 2

    1 fennel bulb, sliced as thinly as possible
    1 navel orange, sectioned
    2 garlic cloves, finely chopped
    2 tablespoons olive oil
    ½ teaspoon sea salt

Combine all the ingredients in a bowl. Toss until well combined and serve.

CAESAR SALAD

Servings: 2

    2 romaine hearts, coarsely chopped
    ½ cup Caesar Dressing (pages 148–149)
    1 handful Sea Kale Chips (page 136)
    1 handful Chive-Miso Flax Crackers (page 134)

In a large bowl toss the romaine with the Caesar Dressing. Top with the Sea Kale Chips and Chive-Miso Flax Crackers.

EVERYDAY RAW SALAD

Servings: 4

    5 cups mixed salad greens
    ½ red onion, thinly sliced
    1 cucumber, peeled, seeded, and sliced
    2 tomatoes, cored and chopped into large rough chunks
    1 red bell pepper, stemmed, seeded, and thinly sliced
    1 carrot, peeled and grated
    ½ cup of your favorite dressing

Place the greens, onion, cucumber, tomatoes, pepper, and carrot in a large bowl. Toss well with the dressing.

BRAD'S FAVORITE SEAWEED SALAD

Servings: 4

DRESSING

   ¼ cup nama shoyu or coconut aminos
   ¼ cup vinegar
   ½ cup sesame oil
   ½ teaspoon ground cloves

SALAD

   2 cups mixed greens
   1 cup dried wakame or arame, soaked for 30 minutes and drained
   ½ cup cucumber, peeled, seeded, and thinly sliced
   ½ cup red bell pepper, stemmed, seeded, and thinly sliced
   2 scallions, ends trimmed and finely chopped
   3 tablespoons minced parsley
   1 apple, peeled, cored, and thinly sliced
   ½ cup dried cherries
   2 tablespoons sesame seeds

Pour the nama shoyu, vinegar, and sesame oil into a mason jar and add the ground cloves. Seal tightly and shake until emulsified. Place the greens, wakame, cucumber, red pepper, scallions, parsley, apple, and cherries in a bowl and toss with the dressing. Sprinkle on the sesame seeds.

TOMATO, AVOCADO, AND BASIL SALAD

Servings: 2

   2 large heirloom tomatoes, cored and sliced into ½-inch rounds
   ½ avocado, peeled, pitted, and sliced lengthwise ½ inch thick
   1 handful basil leaves, torn
   2 tablespoons fresh chives, minced
   1 tablespoon raw balsamic vinegar
   3 tablespoons olive oil
   Sea salt and freshly ground black pepper, to taste

Arrange the tomato and avocado slices on a large plate. Scatter the basil and chives over all. Drizzle with the vinegar and oil, and season with salt and pepper to taste.

DARK LEAFY GREEN SALAD

Servings: 2

3 stalks chard, ribs removed, chopped
3 stalks kale, ribs removed, chopped
1 handful spinach
1 handful arugula
3 tablespoons minced parsley
4 tablespoons of your favorite sprouts
½ cup of your favorite dressing

In a large bowl, combine the chard, kale, spinach, arugula, parsley, and sprouts. Toss with the dressing.

DELI SALAD

Servings: 4

1 cup sunflower seeds, soaked overnight and drained
1 cup raw almonds, soaked overnight and drained
½ cup coarsely chopped celery
½ cup coarsely chopped pickles*
¼ cup coarsely chopped red onion
1 handful fresh dill leaves
½ green apple, cored
2 tablespoons lemon juice
6 tablespoons Raw Mayonnaise (page 144)
2 tablespoons olive oil
1 teaspoon sea salt

Place the sunflower seeds and almonds in a food processor fitted with a steel blade and pulse until coarse. Pour the mixture into a mixing bowl. Place the celery, pickles, onion, dill, and apple in food processor and pulse until ingredients are finely chopped. Add the vegetables and fruit to the nut mixture. Pour the lemon juice, Raw Mayonnaise, olive oil, and sea salt over all and mix well.

Look for preservative-free pickles such as Bubbies brand pickles.

ASIAN COLESLAW SALAD

Servings: 4

DRESSING

    6 tablespoons vinegar
    6 tablespoons sesame oil
    2 tablespoons raw tahini
    2 tablespoons Raw Mayonnaise (page 144)
    2 tablespoons nama shoyu
    5 pitted dates
    1 (1-inch) piece ginger, peeled and minced
    2 garlic cloves
    ½ jalapeño, seeded

SALAD

    1 small head of green or napa cabbage, cored and coarsely chopped
    2 red bell peppers, stems and seeds removed, coarsely chopped
    2 carrots, peeled and coarsely chopped
    6 scallions, ends trimmed and chopped
    ½ cup cilantro, chopped

To make the dressing, pour the vinegar, sesame oil, tahini, Raw Mayonnaise, and nama shoyu into a blender. Add the dates, ginger, garlic, and jalapeño and blend until smooth. For the salad, place the cabbage, peppers, carrots, scallions, and cilantro into a food processor fitted with a steel blade and pulse until finely chopped. Place the vegetable mixture in a bowl and pour the dressing over all. Mix until well combined.

CARROT SALAD

Servings: 4

> 5 carrots, peeled and grated
> 3 tablespoons lemon juice
> 3 tablespoons dried cranberries
> ¼ teaspoon cinnamon
> ¼ small fresh chili pepper, finely chopped
> Pinch of nutmeg
> 1 cup finely chopped fresh mint
> 2 tablespoons pumpkin seeds

Place all the ingredients in a bowl and mix well.

HEMP SEED SALAD

Servings: 2

> 2 tablespoons finely chopped parsley leaves
> 4 tablespoons hemp seeds
> 1 cup sprouted quinoa
> 2 tomatoes, cored and coarsely chopped
> 1 tablespoon chopped chives
> 1 tablespoon lemon juice
> 2 tablespoons olive oil
> Sea salt

Place all the ingredients in a bowl and mix well.

EASY GRATED SALAD

Servings: 4

> 1 cup grated daikon
> 1 cup peeled and grated carrots
> 1 cup grated beets
> 1 bunch cilantro, leaves only
> Grapefruit Star Dressing (page 149) or your favorite dressing

In a bowl, combine the daikon, carrots, beets, and cilantro. Add the dressing and toss well.

MAYAN SALAD

Servings: 4

DRESSING

 2 avocados, peeled, pitted, and cut into chunks
 ¼ cup fresh lime juice
 1 teaspoon chili powder
 ¼ cup extra-virgin olive oil
 2 tablespoons honey
 1 tablespoon cacao powder
 2 tablespoons finely chopped fresh cilantro
 1 garlic clove, peeled and minced
 ½ jalapeño pepper

SALAD

 Kernels from 4 ears of corn
 4 heirloom tomatoes, cored and diced
 ¼ cup diced red bell pepper
 1 head bok choy, sliced thinly
 ½ cup diced Vidalia onion
 ¼ cup thinly sliced radishes

Place all the ingredients for the dressing into a blender and process until smooth. In a bowl mix the corn, tomatoes, red pepper, bok choy, onion, and radishes. Pour the dressing over the vegetables and toss well.

SOUPS

CUCUMBER SOUP WITH AVOCADO AND DILL

Servings: 4

1 medium cucumber, peeled and seeded

1 ripe small avocado, peeled and pitted

1 scallion, ends trimmed

1 garlic clove

2 tablespoons fresh cilantro, divided

2½ tablespoons fresh dill

2 tablespoons fresh lemon juice

½ cup cold water

½ cup ice cubes

1 medium tomato, cored and chopped coarsely

Put the cucumber, avocado, scallion, garlic, cilantro, 1½ tablespoons of the dill, lemon juice, water, and ice cubes into a blender. Puree until smooth. Garnish with chopped tomato and remaining dill.

GAZPACHO

Servings: 4

8 ripe tomatoes, peeled and cored

½ cucumber, peeled, seeded, and coarsely chopped

½ red bell pepper, stemmed, seeded, and coarsely chopped

½ red onion, coarsely chopped

2 garlic cloves

½ cup walnuts, soaked overnight and drained

2 teaspoons sea salt

½ teaspoon cayenne pepper

2 teaspoons raw vinegar

4 tablespoons extra-virgin olive oil

Juice of ½ lemon

Lemon slices, for garnish

Place all of the ingredients except the garnish in a blender or food processor and blend until desired consistency. Serve in tall glasses with a slice of lemon.

RAWKIN' RED BELL PEPPER SOUP

Servings: 2

2 large red bell peppers, stemmed, seeded, and coarsely chopped
1 large carrot, peeled and coarsely chopped
1 medium avocado, peeled, pitted, and coarsely chopped
½ teaspoon sea salt
½ cup purified water
2 tablespoons fresh-squeezed lemon juice
½ cup cashew pieces

Place the red peppers, carrot, avocado, salt, water, and lemon juice in a blender and blend until smooth. Pour into serving bowls and top each with ¼ cup cashew pieces.

ENTREES

BURRITOS

Servings: 2

WALNUT TACO MEAT

    1 cup walnuts

    2 teaspoons cumin

    ¼ teaspoon chili powder

    1 teaspoon sea salt

SALSA

    1 large tomato, cored and diced

    1 cup fresh corn kernels

    ¼ cup chopped red onion

    2 tablespoons chopped cilantro

    1 teaspoon apple cider vinegar

    1 teaspoon sea salt

CASHEW SOUR CREAM

    ½ cup cashews, soaked 4 hours and drained

    1 teaspoon lemon juice

    ½ teaspoon sea salt

THE ASSEMBLY

    4 large collard leaves

    1 avocado, peeled, pitted, and sliced

    Fresh lime wedges, for garnish

    Minced cilantro, for garnish

MAKE THE WALNUT TACO MEAT

Process all the ingredients in a food processor until the mixture is the consistency of cooked ground beef.

MAKE THE SALSA

In a bowl, mix all of the ingredients together and let stand for at least 2 hours.

Make the Cashew Sour Cream
Place all of the ingredients in a food processor and pulse until smooth.

Assemble the Burritos
Overlay 2 collard green leaves together. Layer the Walnut Taco Meat, Salsa, and Cashew Sour Cream and avocado in the middle of greens. Fold in the sides, then fold over the bottom of the collard and roll up the leaves to make a burrito. Repeat with the remaining collard leaves, meat, salsa, sour cream, and avocado. Garnish with lime wedges and minced cilantro.

SOUTH PACIFIC OYSTER MUSHROOMS

Servings: 4

> 1 cup slivered fresh oyster mushrooms
> ½ red onion, minced
> 2 tablespoons grated ginger
> 1 chili pepper, minced
> ½ cup raw vinegar
> 1 tablespoon water
> 1 seedless cucumber, peeled and chopped
> 2 tablespoons sea salt
> 1 tablespoon freshly ground black pepper
> ¼ cup lemon juice

Mix all the ingredients in a bowl. Cover the mixture and marinate in the fridge overnight.

BLT

Servings: 4

> 4 tablespoons Raw Mayonnaise (page 144)
> 8 slices of raw Onion Bread (page 138) or any kind of raw bread, or
>   4 large romaine lettuce leaves
> 12 slices of Eggplant Bacon (page 137)
> 2 tomatoes, cored and sliced into ¼-inch rounds
> 2 avocados, peeled, pitted, and cut lengthwise into ¼-inch slices
> 3 cups sprouts, your choice

Spread the Raw Mayonnaise onto the raw bread. Add three slices of Eggplant Bacon, and tomato, avocado, and sprouts to each sandwich. Top with another slice of bread.

RAW PAD THAI

Servings: 4

DRESSING
   ¼ cup almond butter
   1 tablespoon tahini
   2 tablespoons coconut aminos
   1 tablespoon dulse flakes
   2 garlic cloves
   Pinch cayenne pepper
   8 pitted dates, soaked overnight and drained
   1 tablespoon lime zest
   ¼ cup lime juice
   2 tablespoons sesame oil
   ¼ cup water
   ½ cup crushed cashews

   2 small zucchini, chopped, stem removed
   1 cup sprouts
   2 scallions, ends trimmed and thinly sliced
   1 red bell pepper, stemmed, seeded, and sliced into thick strips
   ½ cup Pickled Red Cabbage (page 141)
   ½ red onion, sliced
   1 handful cilantro leaves, chopped

Place all the ingredients for the dressing into a blender and process until smooth. In a bowl combine the zucchini, sprouts, scallions, red pepper, Pickled Red Cabbage, onion, and cilantro. Pour the dressing over the vegetables and toss well to combine.

LASAGNA ROLLS

Servings: 2; 4 rolls per serving

> 1 medium zucchini, thinly sliced 8 times lengthwise
> 1 tomato, cored and thinly sliced 8 times
> Marinara Sauce (page 153)
> Pesto (page 152)
> Pine Nut Cheese (page 135)

Place a strip of zucchini on a flat surface. Layer a tablespoon each of Marinara, Pesto, and Pine Nut Cheese. Place a slice of tomato on top. Roll up and place seam side down on a platter and top with additional marinara sauce.

KOLOURFUL KABOBS

Servings: 4

> ½ cup coconut aminos
> ½ cup sesame oil
> 1 tablespoon lime zest
> 1 red pepper, stemmed, seeded, and cut into 1-inch pieces
> ½ fresh pineapple, peeled, cored, and chopped into 1-inch chunks
> 2 zucchini, trimmed and chopped into 1-inch chunks
> 1 sweet onion, cut into 1-inch pieces
> 2 cups mushrooms, stemmed and quartered
> Bamboo skewers
> Thai Dream Dressing (pages 147–148) or dressing of your choice

Combine the coconut aminos, sesame oil, and lime zest in a small bowl. Thread the red pepper, pineapple, zucchini, onion, and mushrooms onto the skewers. Brush the kabobs with the coconut aminos mixture and marinate for 30 minutes at room temperature. Serve with dressing and enjoy with a garden salad.

VEGGIE RIBBON NOODLES

Servings: 4

> 2 small zucchini, peeled and spiralized
>
> 6 asparagus, lower ¼ of stem removed, julienned
>
> 2 carrots, peeled and julienned or grated
>
> 1 large red bell pepper, stemmed, seeded, and julienned
>
> 3 scallions, ends trimmed, whites and light green parts only, thinly sliced lengthwise
>
> Pesto (page 152) or your favorite dressing

Gently toss the zucchini, asparagus, carrots, red pepper, and scallions. Top with Pesto or your favorite dressing.

STUFFED MUSHROOMS

Servings: 4

> 12 button mushrooms, cleaned
>
> ½ red or yellow bell pepper, seeded and coarsely chopped
>
> ⅔ cup pine nuts, soaked overnight and drained
>
> 1 garlic clove
>
> 1 packed handful fresh basil leaves
>
> 1 handful fresh spinach
>
> 1 tablespoon lemon juice
>
> ½ teaspoon sea salt
>
> Olive oil

Twist the stems off the mushrooms; set the mushrooms and stems aside. Place the bell pepper in a food processor and pulse until chopped into small pieces; do not puree. Transfer the pepper to a mixing bowl. Place the mushroom stems, pine nuts, garlic, basil, spinach, lemon juice, and salt in the food processor and pulse until blended smooth. Add the mixture to the chopped pepper and mix well. Stuff the mushroom caps with the filling and drizzle with olive oil. The stuffed mushrooms can also be warmed in a dehydrator at 100°F for 6 hours.

BRAD'S "NOT SO" SUSHI ROLLS

Servings: 4

4 tablespoons Pine Nut Cheese (page 135) or Deli Salad (page 156)
4 nori sheets
1 carrot, peeled and julienned
1 cucumber, peeled, seeded, and julienned
1 small bunch of chives, finely chopped
1 avocado, peeled, pitted, and thinly sliced
2 cups sunflower sprouts or pea shoots
1 tablespoon peeled and grated ginger
½ cup nama shoyu
1 teaspoon lemon juice

Spread Pine Nut Cheese or Deli Salad on each nori sheet, then layer the carrots, cucumber, chives, avocado, and ginger on top. Roll up the nori sheets, lengthwise, into long cylinders, and cut into "sushi rolls." Combine the nama shoyu and lemon in a small bowl and serve alongside for dipping.

PORTOBELLO BURGERS

Servings: 4

½ cup extra-virgin olive oil
1 teaspoon vinegar
¼ cup nama shoyu
Pinch salt
2 garlic cloves
4 portobello mushrooms, cleaned and stemmed
4 slices of raw Onion Bread (page 138) or any type of raw bread, or
    4 large lettuce leaves

SUGGESTED TOPPINGS
Sliced tomato
Sliced onion
Sliced avocado
Red bell pepper strips

In a blender combine the oil, vinegar, nama shoyu, salt, and garlic. Blend until emulsified. Brush the portobello caps with the mixture and let sit for 30 minutes. Drain the marinade and serve the mushrooms on raw bread or lettuce leaves with the suggested toppings.

ZUCCHINI PIZZA

Note: This recipe can be made only with a dehydrator. The crust will take the shape of the model dehydrator you use.

Serves 6–8; makes two 13" crusts

7 cups coarsely chopped zucchini
5 garlic cloves
1 cup flaxseeds
4 cups sunflower seeds
¼ cup extra-virgin olive oil
3 tablespoons Pesto (page 152)
1 tablespoon oregano
1 tablespoon sea salt

SUGGESTED TOPPINGS
1½ cups sliced mushrooms, marinated in 2 tablespoons olive oil, 1 tablespoon balsamic vinegar, and 1 teaspoon sea salt for at least 10 minutes
1 cup sliced red and green bell peppers
¼ cup sliced red onion, marinated in 2 tablespoons olive oil, 1 tablespoon balsamic vinegar, and 1 teaspoon sea salt for at least 10 minutes
¼ teaspoon sea salt
1 tablespoon olive oil

Place the zucchini, garlic, flaxseeds, sunflower seeds, olive oil, Pesto, oregano, and sea salt into a blender or food processor and blend until smooth. Spread the mixture onto a dehydrator tray and dehydrate for 10–12 hours, turning over halfway. Remove the crust from the dehydrator and add your choice of toppings: Try the Rawcho Cheese (page 134), Pine Nut Cheese (page 135), Marinara (page 153), or add a bit of Brad's Zingin' Hot Sauce (page 146) if you're feeling spicy!

BBQ VEGGIE BURGERS

Note: This recipe can be made only with a dehydrator.

Servings: 4

- ½ cup pumpkin seeds, soaked overnight and drained
- ½ cup pine nuts, soaked overnight and drained
- ½ cup ground flaxseeds
- 2 tablespoons ground chia seeds
- 2 tablespoons BBQ Sauce (page 145)
- 2 teaspoons lemon juice
- 2 tablespoons extra-virgin olive oil
- 1 garlic clove, minced
- 1 teaspoon cumin
- 1 small onion, chopped coarsely
- 1 carrot, peeled and chopped coarsely
- 1 celery stalk, chopped coarsely
- 10 stalks cilantro

Place the pumpkin seeds, pine nuts, flaxseeds, chia seeds, BBQ Sauce, lemon juice, olive oil, garlic, and cumin in a food processor and blend until the mixture has a partially smooth consistency. Transfer into a mixing bowl.

Place the onion, carrot, celery, and cilantro in a food processor and pulse until finely minced. Add to the seed mixture and mix until thoroughly combined. Line dehydrator trays with parchment paper.

With your hands, form the mixture into ¾-inch-thick patties, similar to burger patties, and place them on the trays. Dehydrate at 115°F for 4 hours. Reduce heat to 100°F, flip the burgers over, and dehydrate for another 4 hours. Once the burger patties are holding together, remove the tray liner and continue dehydrating in the machine until they reach desired consistency.

KIDS' TREATS

FRUIT LEATHER

Note: This recipe can be made only with a dehydrator.

Servings: 6

> 2 cups strawberries, leaves and stems removed
> 3 cups coarsely chopped apples
> 2 cups red grapes

Blend the ingredients in a blender or food processor until smooth. Spread the mixture 1/8 inch thick on teflex sheets and dehydrate at 110°F for 4 hours or until firm. Peel the dried mixture off the tray, cut into strips, and enjoy.

MINI FRUIT BOWLS

Servings: 4

> 1 pineapple, peeled, cored, and chopped into small chunks
> 2 mangoes, peeled, pitted, and chopped into small chunks
> 1 quart strawberries, leaves and stems removed, and sliced in half
> 4 kiwi, peeled and sliced into coins
> 2 cups red grapes

Place all the ingredients in a large bowl and toss gently to combine. Spoon into serving bowls.

MIAH'S ENERGY BALLS

Servings: 16 (2 balls per serving)

> 3 cups ground oat groats*
> 1 cup golden raisins
> 1 cup dried cranberries
> 1 teaspoon sea salt
> 1 tablespoon lucuma powder (optional)
> 1 cup raw cacao powder
> Cinnamon, to taste

1 cup vanilla agave (or plain agave with ½ teaspoon vanilla extract),
   or honey
5 tablespoons coconut oil, gently warmed to melt
1 cup almond butter

Place the ground oats, raisins, cranberries, sea salt, lucuma powder if using, cacao powder, and cinnamon in a blender and blend until combined. Pour the mixture into a large mixing bowl. Add the agave, coconut oil, and almond butter. Mix by hand until the mixture sticks together. Refrigerate for an hour, then remove from fridge and form into bite-size balls and place on a parchment-lined plate. Put the plate in the refrigerator until ready to consume. Or wrap individually and freeze—you can grab before you go!

To grind, place the groats in a blender or food processor and pulse until coarse.

TERIYAKI NORI CRISPS

Note: This recipe can be made only with a dehydrator.

Servings: 4

2 tablespoons nama shoyu
2 tablespoons sesame oil
1 teaspoon raw honey
½ teaspoon garlic powder
½ teaspoon ginger powder
10 nori sheets

To make the teriyaki sauce, pour the nama shoyu, sesame oil, and honey in a blender Add the garlic powder and ginger and blend until smooth. Pour the sauce into a bowl and, using a brush, spread a thin layer of sauce onto each sheet of nori. Dehydrate sheets at 115°F for about 4 hours or until crisp.

BRAZIL NUT MYLK GONE WILD!

Makes 1 quart

> 2 cups water
> 2 cups Brazil nuts, soaked overnight and drained
> 2 teaspoons vanilla agave (or plain agave with ½ teaspoon of vanilla extract)
> 3 bananas
> ½ cup maple syrup
> Dash of sea salt

Place the water, Brazil nuts, vanilla agave, bananas, maple .syrup, and salt in a blender and blend until nuts are liquefied. Strain the mixture through a nut bag. Pour the mixture into glasses or a pitcher. Serve right away or keep chilled. You can freeze this in a popsicle tray for a refreshing treat.

STRAWBERRY MILK

Makes 1 quart

> 1 cup cashews, soaked 4–6 hours and drained
> 1 cup strawberries, leaves and stems removed
> 2 teaspoons raw honey
> 1 teaspoon vanilla extract or seeds from ½ vanilla bean
> 1 tablespoon maca powder
> ½ teaspoon lemon juice
> 2 cups water

Place all the ingredients in a blender and blend until smooth. Strain the mixture through a nut bag into glasses or a pitcher. Serve immediately or keep chilled. Discard the solids.

CHOCOLATE FRUIT AND NUT BAR

Servings: 4

> 1 cup cacao butter (I recommend Navitas Naturals brand), melted on low heat
> 1 cup macadamia nuts, soaked overnight and drained
> ½ cup maple syrup

2 tablespoons maca powder
½ cup goji berries
⅓ cup cacao nibs

Place the cacao butter, macadamia nuts, maple syrup, and maca powder in a blender and blend until smooth. Pour the mixture on a sheet pan and spread evenly. Sprinkle with goji berries and/or cacao nibs. Chill in the refrigerator until firm, at least 1 hour.

BRAD'S FROZEN GREEN SMOOTHIE POPS

Servings: 8

¾ cup kale juice (approximately 3 leaves, juiced)
¼ cup parsley juice (approximately 1 cup packed parsley leaves, juiced)
1½ cups chopped pineapple
1 small banana
1 cup coconut water
1 tablespoon lime juice
½ teaspoon dulse flakes

Place all the ingredients in a blender or food processor and blend until smooth. Pour the mixture into popsicle molds and freeze overnight.

BRAD'S RAW MAC AND CHEESE

Servings: 4

2 cups packaged kelp noodles (found in health food stores) or julienned zucchini, carrots, or jicama.
1 cup Rawcho Cheese (page 134)

Place the noodles or veggies in a mixing bowl, add the Rawcho Cheese, and mix well. To warm the recipe, pour it in a bowl and place it in a dehydrator with trays removed at 115°F for 1 hour.

FUDGSICLES

Servings: 12

> 3 frozen bananas, peeled and chopped into chunks
> 1½ cups coconut milk (I recommend Native Forest Organic
>   Coconut Milk brand)
> 3 heaping tablespoons raw cacao powder
> ¼ avocado, peeled and pitted
> 8 pitted dates
> 1 teaspoon vanilla
> ¼ teaspoon sea salt

Place all the ingredients in a blender and blend until smooth. Pour the mixture into popsicle molds and freeze until firm.

DESSERTS

MANGO MOUSSE

Servings: 4

> 2 cups diced mango
> 1 cup coconut oil
> Pinch salt

Blend the mango in a blender until liquefied. Add the coconut oil and salt and blend a bit more. Chill in a bowl for 4 or more hours. Spoon into dessert dishes and enjoy.

ORANGE VANILLA MACAROONS

Servings: 6–8

> 3 cups unsweetened shredded raw coconut
> ¾ cup raw agave or local raw honey
> ½ cup fresh orange juice
> 1 tablespoon orange zest
> Pinch salt

Place all the ingredients in a food processor and pulse until fully incorporated. Scoop the mixture out by tablespoons and press into small mounds. Place the cookies on a plate and refrigerate until firm.

CHIA CHAI PUDDING

Servings: 4

> 2 cups nut or coconut milk
> 1½ teaspoons ground cardamom
> ½ teaspoon cinnamon
> ¼ teaspoon ground cloves
> ¼ teaspoon nutmeg
> 1 teaspoon vanilla extract
> 3 tablespoons maple syrup
> ¼–½ cup chia seeds
> Handful fruit, to garnish

Blend milk, cardamom, cinnamon, cloves, nutmeg, vanilla, and maple syrup together in a blender on high speed until smooth. Place the chia seeds in a bowl and pour the mixture over the seeds. Stir thoroughly with a whisk or a fork. Let it sit for 5 minutes, then stir again. Let it sit another 10 minutes, then stir again. Refrigerate the pudding overnight and check in the morning for desired consistency. If it's too thick, add more milk.

PAPAYA PUDDING

Servings: 4

> 1 papaya, peeled, seeded, and coarsely chopped
> 1 small avocado, peeled, pitted, and quartered
> 1 cup baby spinach

Place all the ingredients in a blender and process for about 30 seconds until smooth. Refrigerate for an hour to thicken before serving.

RAW CHOCOLATE CHIP COOKIES

Makes about 6 cookies

CHOCOLATE CHIPS
> ½ cup coconut oil
> ½ cup carob powder
> ½ cup raw cacao

COOKIE DOUGH
> ¾ cup ground oat groats*
> ¼ cup agave nectar
> 2 teaspoons vanilla extract
> ½ cup coconut oil, melted
> 1¾ cups almond flour, plus additional for finishing

MAKE THE CHOCOLATE CHIPS
Place the oil, carob, and cacao in a bowl and mix until well combined. Spread the mixture on a plate and place it in the freezer until it's firm, at least 1 hour. Remove the chocolate mixture from the plate and break or chop it into small chunks.

MAKE THE COOKIES

In a large bowl, mix the ground oat groats, agave nectar, vanilla, coconut oil, and almond flour. Fold in the chocolate chips. Form the dough into balls about 1 inch in diameter, roll them in a bit of additional almond flour, and refrigerate for at least 30 minutes before serving.

To grind, place the groats in a blender or food processor and pulse until coarse.

LIME COCONUT CHEESECAKE

Servings: 6

CRUST

> 1½ cups walnuts or pecans, soaked overnight and drained
> 10 pitted dates
> 4 dried apricots
> ¼ teaspoon sea salt
> 1 teaspoon maca powder

FILLING

> 3 cups cashews, soaked for 2–6 hours and drained
> ½ cup raw honey
> ¾ cup coconut oil, melted
> 2 teaspoons vanilla extract
> 6 tablespoons lime juice
> 2 tablespoons lime zest

MAKE THE CRUST

Place the walnuts or pecans, dates, apricots, sea salt, and maca powder in a food processor and pulse to combine. Scoop out the dough and push it into the bottom of an 8-inch pie plate. Put the plate in the fridge while making the filling.

MAKE THE FILLING

Place the cashews, honey, coconut oil, vanilla, lime juice, and lime zest in a blender and puree until smooth. Remove the crust from the refrigerator and pour in the filling. Freeze for at least 4 hours to set. When ready to eat, cut the pie into slices and let them defrost at room temperature for 20 minutes before enjoying.

RAW BERRY CRISP À LA BRAD

Servings: 8

 6 cups mixed berries
 1 tablespoon maple syrup
 1 cup pecans, soaked overnight and drained
 ½ cup walnuts, soaked overnight and drained
 ½ cup pitted dates, coarsely chopped
 1 teaspoon cinnamon

In a 7 x 11-inch dish, toss the berries with the maple syrup. Place the pecans, walnuts, dates, and cinnamon in a food processor and pulse until coarsely ground. Scatter the nut mixture over the berries and serve immediately, or chill until ready to serve.

RAW CUPCAKES

Makes 4 cupcakes

 ¾ cup macadamia nuts, soaked overnight and drained
 ¾ cup pecans, soaked overnight and drained
 5 pitted dates
 3 tablespoons cocoa or carob powder
 2 tablespoons raw honey
 ¼ teaspoon sea salt
 ½ cup unsweetened coconut flakes

FROSTING
 1 avocado, peeled, pitted, and coarsely chopped
 1 tablespoon coconut oil, softened
 2 tablespoons cocoa powder
 2 tablespoons raw honey
 ½ teaspoon vanilla extract

Place the macadamia nuts, pecans, dates, cocoa powder, honey, and salt in a food processor and pulse until well incorporated. In a muffin tin, sprinkle about a teaspoon of coconut into four of the molds, then press equal portions of the mixture into the molds. Refrigerate for at least 1 hour, then pop the cupcakes out of the muffin tin.

Meanwhile, place the avocado, coconut oil, cocoa powder, honey, and vanilla in a food processor and blend until smooth. Dollop the frosting on top of the cupcakes. Chill for another hour and enjoy!

FAVORITE BIRTHDAY CAKE

Servings: 4

2 cups raisins
2 cups cashews, soaked for 1 hour and drained
1 cup pitted dates
Juice from ½ lemon
Blueberries and raspberries, for garnish

For the base, blend the raisins, cashews, and 3–4 dates in the food processor. On a plate form the mixture into a cake shape. Blend the remaining dates and lemon juice and spread the mixture over the cake. Decorate with blueberries, raspberries, or your favorite fruit.

Happy birthday to you!

BUTTER PECAN ICE CREAM

Makes 1 quart

Note: Young coconuts are much more expensive than the older brown ones you usually find in stores, so consider this recipe a special treat. You'll need about three coconuts to make this recipe.

1 cup coconut water, drained from a young coconut
1½ cups nut milk
1 cup chopped young coconut meat
3 tablespoons coconut oil
½ cup raw honey
1 teaspoon vanilla extract or seeds from ½ vanilla bean
1 cup crushed Craic Nuts (page 136)

Place all the ingredients except for the Craic Nuts in a blender and blend until smooth. Stir in the Craic Nuts. Freeze the mixture in an ice cream maker according to the manufacturer's instructions.

MAYAN CHOCOLATE TRUFFLES

Servings: 4

> 1 cup cashew butter
> 1 cup raw honey
> ¾ cup cacao or carob powder, plus additional for finishing
> 1 teaspoon vanilla extract or seeds from ½ vanilla bean
> 1 teaspoon sea salt
> ¼ teaspoon cayenne pepper*
> ½ teaspoon cinnamon
> 2 teaspoons maca powder

Place the cashew butter, honey, cacao, vanilla, salt, cayenne, cinnamon, and maca in a food processor and pulse until well incorporated. Place the additional cacao on a plate. Roll the dough into balls about 1 inch in diameter and then roll them in the cacao. Store the truffles in the refrigerator until ready to serve.

*If you'd like more kick, up this to ½ teaspoon. Spicy!

PECAN SPICE DELIGHT COOKIES

Servings: 6

> 1½ cups raw pecans
> ½ cup unsweetened shredded or desiccated dried coconut
> 1 teaspoon fresh chopped ginger
> ½ teaspoon cinnamon
> Pinch of sea salt
> ½ teaspoon vanilla extract
> ¼ cup raisins
> ¼ cup dried cranberries
> 10–12 pitted dates (use 10 if they are big, 12 if they are small)

Place the pecans, coconut, ginger, cinnamon, salt, and vanilla in a food processor and blend until just incorporated. Add the raisins, cranberries, and dates and continue processing until the mixture begins to stick together when pressed between your fingers. Roll the mixture into balls about 1 inch in diameter. Refrigerate until ready to eat.

CHOCOLATE CHERRY COOKIES

Servings: 6

CHERRY JAM

> 2 cups dried cherries
> ½ cup water
> 2 tablespoons agave nectar
> 1 tablespoon lucuma powder

COOKIES

> 1 cup almond meal left over from making nut milk (page 124)
> 2 cups coarsely chopped pitted dates
> ½ cup cacao powder
> 5 tablespoons coconut oil
> 1 teaspoon cinnamon
> 4 tablespoons hemp seeds
> 1 cup finely shredded dried unsweetened coconut
> 4 tablespoons honey

MAKE THE CHERRY JAM

Place the dried cherries, water, agave, and lucuma powder in a blender and blend until the mixture reaches the consistency of jelly, about 30–60 seconds.

MAKE THE COOKIES

Place all the ingredients in a food processor and pulse until smooth. Roll the cookie dough into 2-inch balls and place them on a cookie sheet. Make an indentation in the middle of each ball. Add a spoonful of Cherry Jam.

TROPICAL GELATO

Makes 1 quart

> 1 cup coconut water
> 1 frozen banana, peeled and chopped into chunks
> 1 cup mango chunks
> 1 cup chopped fresh pineapple
> ¼ cup fresh orange juice
> 2 tablespoons raw honey

1 teaspoon lime juice
¼ teaspoon sea salt

Place all the ingredients in a blender and blend until smooth. Pour the mixture into a plastic or paper container and freeze for at least 6 hours, stirring once or twice during the initial freezing, and then freeze overnight. Alternatively, you can add all the ingredients to an ice cream maker and process according to the manufacturer's instructions.

CHOCOLATE MOUSSE PIE

Servings: 4

CRUST
1 cup almonds, soaked overnight and drained
1 cup pitted dates
½ teaspoon sea salt

MOUSSE
1 cup coconut oil
½ cup raw cacao butter
1 ripe avocado, peeled and pitted
½ cup raw cacao powder
1 cup room temperature coconut oil
½ cup raw honey
½ teaspoon sea salt

MINT SAUCE
¼ cup coconut milk (I recommend Native Forest Organic Coconut Milk)
4–6 fresh mint leaves
½ tablespoon raw honey

TOPPING
2 cups raspberries

MAKE THE CRUST
Place all the ingredients in a food processor and pulse until well incorporated. Press the mixture into an even layer in a 9-inch pie plate. Refrigerate for 1 hour.

MAKE THE MOUSSE

Place all the ingredients in a food processor and pulse until smooth. Pour the mixture into the pie crust and return it to the refrigerator. Refrigerate overnight.

MAKE THE MINT SAUCE

Place all the ingredients in a blender and puree until smooth.

FINISH AND TOPPING

Remove the pie from the refrigerator. Pour the Mint Sauce evenly over the top, arrange the raspberries in a lovely pattern, and chill for at least another 4 hours. Slice and enjoy!

COOKED FOODS

All of these grains benefit from being soaked overnight and drained before cooking. In addition, they can be toasted in a hot pan before cooking to bring out a delicious nutty flavor. All of them are gluten free.

- Brown rice—any variety is good: short, long, or basmati
- Wild rice—this is actually the seed of an aquatic grass
- Quinoa—a seed from the Andes; rinse before use to remove the bitter saponin coating
- Amaranth—a staple of the Aztecs
- Millet—a common grain of India and Africa
- Buckwheat—lovely when toasted

SPICED BASMATI PILAF

Servings: 6

2 cups basmati rice
2 tablespoons sesame oil
2 tablespoons coconut oil
1 small onion, finely chopped
2 garlic cloves, minced
1 tablespoon ground cardamom
1 teaspoon ground coriander
1 teaspoon cinnamon
¼ teaspoon ground fennel seed
½ teaspoon ground ginger
4 cups vegetable broth or water
1 bay leaf
1 carrot, peeled and diced
Sea salt, to taste
2 cups fresh green peas

Pour the rice into a fine mesh strainer and rinse it under cold water until the water runs clear. Place the rice in a pot, cover it with cold water, and let it soak for 30 minutes. Drain the rice, return it to the pot, and set aside.

Over medium heat, heat the sesame and coconut oils in a large saucepan. Add the onion, stir, and cook until softened. Add garlic and sauté for about 1 minute. Add the cardamom, coriander, cinnamon, fennel seed, and ginger, and sauté for another minute. Add the rice and sauté until the rice is translucent and golden brown. Add the broth, bay leaf, carrot, and salt, and bring to a boil. Reduce heat and simmer, partly covered, for about 10 minutes or until rice is cooked to desired tenderness. Add the peas, stir to incorporate, and allow the pilaf to sit for at least 10 minutes before serving.

BRAD'S FAVORITE VEGETARIAN LASAGNA

Servings: 4

- 2 tablespoons extra-virgin olive oil
- 2 tablespoons minced garlic
- 4 cups chopped mixed vegetables: zucchini, mushrooms, broccoli, peppers—anything you like
- 2 cups chopped tomatoes
- 1 cup cooked chickpeas
- 1 teaspoon fresh or dried herbs, such as basil, parsley, and oregano
- 4 large sweet potatoes, peeled and thinly sliced
- 3 tablespoons apple cider vinegar
- ½ teaspoon nutmeg
- ½ teaspoon cinnamon

Preheat the oven to 300°F. In a pan heat the olive oil and sauté the garlic. Add the chopped mixed vegetables and sauté until tender. Add the tomatoes and chickpeas, and cook until the tomatoes are softened. Add the herbs and cook for 5 minutes more. Place half of the sautéed vegetables in a 9 x 12-inch baking dish. Cover with sliced sweet potatoes, then spread the remaining vegetables on top. Cover and bake for 30 minutes. Increase the temperature to 400°F. Remove the cover and cook for 20 minutes more or until crisp on top.

ASIAN PAN-SEARED OYSTER MUSHROOMS AND BABY BOK CHOY WITH MILLET POLENTA

Servings: 4

ASIAN COCONUT SAUCE

⅓ cup coconut milk

1 teaspoon cayenne pepper

1 teaspoon lime juice

1 tablespoon umeboshi vinegar

1 tablespoon nama shoyu

1 tablespoon raw honey

1 cup millet, rinsed well

3 cups vegetable broth or water

1 half head cauliflower, core removed and cut into chunks

Sea salt, to taste

3 tablespoons coconut oil

1 cup oyster mushrooms, thickly sliced

1 tablespoon minced peeled ginger

2 cups baby bok choy, base trimmed, or regular bok choy
    cut into large pieces

3 garlic cloves, minced

½ cup macadamia nuts, soaked overnight and drained

3 tablespoons extra-virgin olive oil

Prepare the Asian Coconut Sauce: In a bowl combine the coconut milk, cayenne, lime juice, vinegar, nama shoyu, and honey. Whisk together and set aside.

Combine the millet, broth, and cauliflower in a large pot and add salt to taste. Bring to a rapid boil, reduce heat, cover, and simmer for 30 minutes or until the cauliflower is soft and the millet is cooked. Remove the pot from the heat and set aside to let cool slightly.

Meanwhile, in a large skillet, heat the coconut oil over medium-high heat. Add the mushrooms and sauté for 2 minutes until all sides are golden brown. Add the ginger and bok choy and sauté for an additional 2–3 minutes until the bok choy is tender. Stir in the Asian Coconut Sauce, bring to a boil, and simmer for a minute.

Place the millet and cauliflower broth, the garlic, macadamia nuts, and olive oil in a food processor and blend until creamy.

Serve the mushrooms and vegetables with sauce over the millet mash.

SUPER QUINOA AND KALE SALAD

Servings: 4

> 3 medium garlic cloves, minced
> 1 tablespoon extra-virgin olive oil
> 1 cup quinoa, rinsed well
> ½ teaspoon ground cumin
> Pinch cayenne pepper
> 1 teaspoon sea salt
> 2 cups water
> ½ bunch Tuscan kale,* ribs removed, and cut into thin strips
> ½ cup Baby Basil Dressing (page 147)

Over medium heat, sauté garlic in olive oil for 30 seconds. Add quinoa and stir to coat. Add cumin and cayenne and heat for 30 seconds. Add salt and water.

Cover and bring to a boil. Reduce heat and simmer, covered, for 15–20 minutes. Remove the pan from the burner and allow the mixture to stand uncovered for 10 minutes, then transfer it to a bowl.

Massage the kale with the dressing, and add dressed kale to the cooled quinoa. Serve chilled or at room temperature.

Also known as lacinato or dinosaur kale.

HONEY ROASTED ROOT VEGETABLES

Servings: 4

> 2 tablespoons raw honey
> 2 tablespoons stone-ground mustard
> 2 tablespoons coconut oil
> 2 tablespoons extra-virgin olive oil
> ½ teaspoon sea salt

1 teaspoon ground coriander

1 sweet potato, peeled and cut into thick sticks

2 turnips, peeled and cut into thick sticks

1 rutabaga, peeled and cut into thick sticks

4 carrots, peeled and cut into thick slices

Preheat oven to 375°F. In a large bowl, whisk together the honey, mustard, oils, salt, and coriander. Add the vegetables to the bowl and massage them with the honey-mustard mixture. Spread the mixture on an unoiled sheet pan and roast for about 30 minutes or until golden brown.

MEDITERRANEAN CHICKPEA STEW

Servings: 4

2 tablespoons extra-virgin olive oil

2 garlic cloves, finely chopped

1 medium yellow onion, diced

1 green bell pepper, cored, seeded, and diced

4 medium zucchini, diced

2 cups coarsely chopped tomatoes

1½ cups chickpeas

1 tablespoon capers

½ teaspoon sea salt

Freshly ground black pepper, to taste

4 cups cooked brown rice

Heat the oil over medium heat in a large skillet. Lower the heat, add the garlic and onions, and cook for 5 minutes until translucent.

Add the green peppers and cook for 5 minutes more. Add the zucchini and cook for 15 minutes, then add the tomatoes. Bring to a simmer and cook for another 20 minutes, or until the zucchini is soft and translucent but still holds its shape. Stir in the chickpeas and capers and cook for another 5 minutes. Season with salt and pepper and serve over brown rice.

ZUCCHINI CHICKPEA CURRY

Servings: 4

2 tablespoons extra-virgin olive oil, divided
1 zucchini, diced
1 yellow squash, diced
1 medium onion, coarsely chopped
3 garlic cloves, crushed
½ teaspoon mustard seed
1 teaspoon ground turmeric
1 teaspoon ground cumin
1 teaspoon ground coriander
1 teaspoon chili powder
1 teaspoon sea salt
1 cup diced tomatoes
1 cup cooked chickpeas
1 cup vegetable broth

Heat 1 tablespoon of the oil in a large skillet or wok over medium-high heat. Sauté the zucchini and yellow squash. Set aside. Using the same pan, heat the remaining 1 tablespoon of oil over medium heat. Cook the onion, garlic, and mustard seed in oil for 3–5 minutes, or until the onion is soft. Season with the ground turmeric, cumin, coriander, chili powder, and salt. Mix in the tomatoes, then stir in the zucchini and squash, chickpeas, and vegetable broth. Bring to a boil, reduce heat to medium low, and simmer for 15 minutes.

BLACK BEAN PATTIES

Servings: 4

2 tablespoons olive oil
2 shallots, minced
2 garlic cloves, minced
½ teaspoon ground cumin
½ teaspoon ground coriander
½ cup corn
½ teaspoon sea salt

2 sun-dried tomatoes, minced

½ carrot, peeled and grated

2 cups cooked black beans

½ cup cooked brown rice

1 tablespoon chopped parsley

1 tablespoon dulse flakes

Heat the oil in a skillet over medium heat and sauté the shallots and garlic until they are softened. Add the cumin, coriander, corn, and salt and sauté for 2 more minutes. Pour the mixture into a bowl and add the tomatoes, carrots, beans, rice, parsley, and dulse flakes. Mix all together with a potato masher until well incorporated. Form the mixture into 4 balls and press each ball into a patty.

Heat a clean skillet to medium-high heat, add a couple tablespoons of olive oil, and sauté the patties until they are browned on each side. Serve with salad or on sprouted buns with your favorite toppings.

VEGETABLE NAPOLEON

Servings: 4

1 large sweet potato, peeled and cut lengthwise into 8 slices

8 portobello mushrooms, cleaned, stemmed, and gills removed

1 zucchini, sliced lengthwise

1 large tomato, stem removed, cut into 8 even slices

¼ cup extra-virgin olive oil, plus more for drizzling

Sea salt and freshly ground black pepper, to taste

Lemon zest

8 sprigs fresh basil or Pesto (page 152)

Preheat oven to 325°F. Bring a pot of water to a boil, then add the sweet potato. Boil for 5 minutes, then remove the slices and drain in a colander. Once they are cool, pat them dry. On an oiled sheet pan, lay out the mushrooms, zucchini, tomatoes, and sweet potato. Drizzle the vegetables with ¼ cup olive oil, and sprinkle with salt, pepper, and lemon zest. Bake them in the oven for 20 minutes. Remove the pan from the oven and let cool until you can pick up the veggies comfortably.

To assemble the napoleons, place the mushrooms on a serving plate. Top each with a slice of zucchini, then sweet potato and tomato. Finish with a drizzle of olive oil and basil leaves or a dollop of Pesto.

JACKET SWEET POTATO

Servings: 4

> 4 sweet potatoes, washed and pricked with a fork several times
> ¼ cup extra-virgin olive oil
> 1 tablespoon sea salt
> 1 tablespoon coconut oil, melted
> Sea Kale Chips or Craic Nuts (page 136), for garnish

Preheat oven to 375°F. Rub the sweet potatoes with olive oil and salt. Bake for 60–75 minutes, depending on the size of the sweet potatoes. Split open the potatoes and drizzle with the coconut oil, then dress them with a topping such as Sea Kale Chips or Craic Nuts.

CRISPY ZUCCHINI AND CHICKPEA HERB SALAD

Servings: 4

DRESSING
> 1 small red onion, finely sliced
> 1 jalapeño, seeded and thinly sliced
> 4 tablespoons lemon juice
> 6 tablespoons extra-virgin olive oil
> ½ teaspoon sea salt
> ¼ teaspoon freshly ground black pepper

> 2 cups cooked chickpeas
> 4 tablespoons sunflower oil
> 1 zucchini, cut in half lengthwise and sliced ½-inch thick
> ½ cup chopped mint
> ½ cup chopped fresh green or purple basil
> 1 handful of your favorite sprouts
> Pine Nut Cheese (page 135)
> Additional mint and basil, chopped, for garnish

To make the dressing, whisk the onion, jalapeño, lemon juice, olive oil, salt, and pepper until well incorporated. Stir the chickpeas into the dressing and let marinate for 10 minutes.

Heat the sunflower oil in a skillet over medium-high heat. Fry the zucchini slices in small batches, without overcrowding, until they are lightly browned on one or both sides. In a large bowl, place the mint, basil, and sprouts and toss with the chickpeas and dressing. Divide the salad among four plates and top with the hot zucchini slices. Serve with a dollop of Pine Nut Cheese and garnish with herbs on top.

BAKED BUTTERNUTOPIA

Servings: 4

    1 butternut squash, halved and seeds removed
    ¼ cup extra-virgin olive oil, plus additional for finishing
    1 red onion, finely chopped
    1 garlic clove, finely chopped
    1 teaspoon ground coriander
    Pinch cayenne pepper
    2 tablespoons fresh thyme leaves
    ½ cup diced shiitake mushrooms
    5 sun-dried tomatoes, finely chopped
    Sea salt and freshly ground black pepper, to taste
    1 cup cooked brown rice or quinoa
    ½ cup sunflower seeds, lightly toasted

Preheat oven to 425°F. Using a spoon, scoop out about a cup of squash from each half to make a trench and chop it up. Add the chopped squash to a skillet with the olive oil, onion, garlic, coriander, cayenne, thyme, shiitake mushrooms, and sun-dried tomatoes. Sauté for about 5 minutes, or until softened, and add salt and pepper to taste. Stir in the rice and sunflower seeds, stuff the mixture into the 2 halves of the squash, then press them together. Rub the skin of the squash with a little olive oil, wrap it in aluminum foil, and bake in the preheated oven for about 1½ hours. To serve, carefully peel off the aluminum foil and guide a knife down between the two halves. Garnish with additional fresh thyme.

SPAGHETTI SQUASH BROCCOLI ALFREDO

Servings: 4

1 spaghetti squash, cut in half and seeds scraped out
1 large head broccoli, cut into small florets
1 cup Macadamia Alfredo Sauce (page 152)
1 cup fresh basil leaves, torn

Preheat oven to 375°F. Place the squash halves cut side down in a baking dish and bake for 40 minutes. Meanwhile, bring 2 quarts of water to a boil in a saucepan. Blanch broccoli for 3 minutes and then drain it in a colander. Remove the dish from the oven and set it aside until the squash is cool enough to handle. Scoop the squash flesh out with a fork to form "spaghetti," and place it in a mixing bowl. Mix the squash, broccoli, and Macadamia Alfredo Sauce together and serve with a sprinkle of basil leaves.

ORIENTAL STIR-FRY

Servings: 4

4 tablespoons sesame oil
1 garlic clove, minced
1 (1-inch) piece ginger, peeled and grated
3 scallions, ends trimmed and thinly sliced diagonally
1 cup mushrooms, cleaned and sliced
1 cup sugar snap peas, sliced
1 cup finely sliced red cabbage
1 carrot, peeled and grated
1 cup mung bean sprouts
1 teaspoon cinnamon
½ teaspoon ground cloves
½ teaspoon freshly ground black pepper
2 teaspoons raw vinegar
1 teaspoon maple syrup
2 teaspoons nama shoyu
1 tablespoon Spirulina Seaweed Gomasio (page 144)
Sesame seeds, for garnish
Cilantro leaves, for garnish

Heat the sesame oil in a skillet or a wok over medium-high heat. Cook the garlic, ginger, and scallions for 1 minute. Add in the mushrooms and sauté for 3–5 minutes until browned. Add the peas, cabbage, carrot, and sprouts and cook for another 2 minutes or until vegetables soften. Add cinnamon, cloves, pepper, vinegar, maple syrup, and nama shoyu. Increase the heat to high for 30 seconds, then remove from the heat and spoon the stir-fry into a serving bowl. Plate and sprinkle with Spirulina Seaweed Gomasio, sesame seeds, and cilantro leaves. Serve with cooked grain, such as quinoa, brown rice, or millet.

THAI EGGPLANT CURRY

Servings: 4

> 6 tablespoons sesame oil
> 2 eggplants, peeled and cut into bite-sized pieces
> 1 red bell pepper, stemmed, seeded, and julienned
> 1 scallion, ends trimmed and finely sliced
> 3 garlic cloves, minced
> 1 (1-inch) piece ginger, peeled and grated
> 3 tablespoons finely chopped cilantro
> 1 jalapeño, seeded and minced
> 1 teaspoon ground coriander
> 2 cups whole coconut milk
> 2 tablespoons lime zest
> 1 tablespoon lemon zest
> 1 tablespoon nama shoyu
> 1 handful fresh basil leaves, torn
> Lime wedges for garnish

Over medium-high heat, heat sesame oil in a wok or large skillet. Add the eggplant and sauté until golden. Add the red pepper, scallion, garlic, ginger, cilantro, jalapeño, and coriander, and cook for 3 minutes. Add the coconut milk, zests, and nama shoyu. Cook on low heat until all the vegetables soften. Garnish with basil leaves and lime wedges. Serve over your favorite cooked grain.

BAKED ARTICHOKE ITALIANO

Servings: 4

> 8 artichokes
> ½ cup extra-virgin olive oil
> 3 tablespoons vinegar
> ½ teaspoon sea salt
> 1 tablespoon dulse flakes
> ½ teaspoon freshly ground black pepper
> 2 tablespoons chopped fresh oregano
> 2 tablespoons chopped fresh parsley
> 2 cups cooked grain, such as rice, quinoa, millet, or wild rice
> 2 cups cherry tomatoes, chopped coarsely
> Additional oregano and parsley, chopped, to finish

Slice the top inch off the artichokes and remove the tough outer leaves. Fill a large pot with several inches of water, and add the artichokes. Cover, and steam the artichokes for 45 minutes. (You can rub them with lemon juice to prevent browning.)

While the artichokes are cooking, whisk together the olive oil, vinegar, salt, dulse, pepper, oregano, and parsley. Place the grain and tomatoes in a bowl and pour the dressing over them. Mix well.

Remove the artichokes from the pot and turn them upside down to drain. When they have cooled to the touch, use a spoon to scoop out the prickly chokes in the center while leaving the tender heart underneath.

Stuff each artichoke heart with the grain and tomato mixture. Serve with a sprinkle of minced fresh herbs on top.

TEMPEH HOLY MOLE

Servings: 4

Mole

> 4 cups vegetable broth or water
> ½ cup sesame or almond oil, divided
> 3 large dried ancho chiles
> 2 tablespoons nama shoyu
> 4 garlic cloves, minced

½ cup raisins

4 tablespoons sesame seeds

2 tablespoons pumpkin seeds

2 teaspoons ground cumin

1 teaspoon chipotle powder

½ teaspoon ground coriander

½ teaspoon ground cloves

½ teaspoon fennel seeds

1 teaspoon salt

½ cup almond butter

½ cup peanut butter

3 tomatoes, cored and diced

4 tablespoons cacao powder

2 teaspoons cinnamon

TEMPEH

4 tablespoons sunflower oil

4 (8-ounce) packs tempeh, cut into triangles

2 cups water

1 teaspoon sea salt

Sesame seeds, for garnish

Sliced scallions, for garnish

MAKE THE MOLE

In a pot, heat the broth. Heat 2 tablespoons of the oil in a large skillet over medium-high heat and sauté the chiles for 2 minutes on each side. Transfer the chiles to the pot of hot broth and allow them to steep for 30 minutes. Remove the chiles with a strainer, remove the stems, slice them open, and discard the seeds. Reserve the liquid. Place the chiles in a blender with the nama shoyu. In the skillet, with the remaining oil over medium heat, sauté the garlic, raisins, sesame and pumpkin seeds, cumin, chipotle, coriander, cloves, fennel seeds, and salt for about 3 minutes. Pour the mixture into the blender with 2 cups of the chile-soaking liquid and puree until smooth. Add the mixture to the pot of remaining liquid and whisk together. Mix in the almond butter, peanut butter, tomatoes, cacao powder, and cinnamon. Bring it to a boil, then reduce heat and simmer for 30 minutes with lid slightly ajar.

Tempeh and Assembly

In a clean skillet, fry the tempeh triangles in oil over medium-high heat, until lightly browned on both sides. Add the water and salt to the pan and bring it to a boil. Cover, reduce the heat, and simmer for 8 minutes. Drain the tempeh and return it to the pan. Pour in the mole and bring to a simmer. Simmer, covered, for 15 minutes. Serve with a sprinkle of sesame seeds and sliced scallions.

ROASTED BUTTERNUT SQUASH SOUP

Servings: 6

4 cups peeled, chopped butternut squash
1 cup fresh apple juice
1/3 cup orange juice
1/3 cup vegetable broth or water
2 large celery stalks
1 teaspoon cinnamon
1/2 teaspoon nutmeg
4 pitted dates
1 teaspoon sea salt
Dash soy sauce

Preheat oven to 350°F. Roast the butternut squash for 30 minutes. Remove from oven and let cool for 15 minutes. Place squash, apple juice, orange juice, vegetable broth, celery stalks, cinnamon, nutmeg, dates, sea salt, and soy sauce in a high-powered blender. Blend until mixture reaches a smooth soup consistency.

TRUFFLED MUSHROOM SOUP

Servings: 6

1/2 cup dried shiitake mushrooms
1/4 cup extra-virgin olive oil
1 pound mixed fresh mushrooms, stemmed and
    sliced
2 garlic cloves, finely sliced
2 shallots, peeled and finely chopped

1 teaspoon fresh thyme leaves

1 teaspoon sea salt

¼ teaspoon freshly ground black pepper

1 quart vegetable broth (page 200) or water

1 handful parsley leaves, finely chopped

2 tablespoons Cashew Sour Cream (pages 162–163)

Juice of ½ lemon

1 teaspoon white truffle oil*

Place the dried shiitake mushrooms in a small bowl, pour 1 cup of boiling water over them, and let soak for at least 20 minutes. After the shiitake are reconstituted, strain them, reserving the liquid, and chop up coarsely. Heat a soup pot over medium-high heat, add the olive oil, and sauté the mushrooms for several minutes, stirring frequently. Add the garlic, shallots, and thyme, reduce heat to medium, and add the salt and pepper. When the shallots begin to soften, add the reserved shiitake liquid and cook until the moisture evaporates. Add vegetable broth, bring to a boil, then reduce heat once more and simmer for about 20 minutes. Remove half the soup from the pot and puree it in a blender, then pour it back in the pot. Add the parsley and Cashew Sour Cream and the lemon juice and stir to combine. Garnish with several drops of truffle oil.

Available in the condiment or oil section in most grocery stores or specialty shops.

MISO SOUP

Servings: 6

1½ quarts water

2 pieces kombu

4 tablespoons dulse flakes

4 fresh shiitake mushrooms, stems removed

1 carrot, peeled and sliced into coins

1 (1-inch) piece ginger, peeled and grated

1 bunch scallions, white parts only, thinly sliced

2 tablespoons chopped cilantro

3 cups fresh spinach, kale, arugula, or other greens of your choice

2 cups yellow miso paste

Nama shoyu, to taste

In a soup pot bring the water to a boil and add the kombu, dulse, and mushrooms. Reduce heat and simmer for 20 minutes. Remove the mushrooms, chop them up, and return them to the pot. Increase heat to bring the soup to a boil, add in the carrots and ginger, and reduce heat once again and simmer for 15 minutes. Add scallions, cilantro, and greens and cook for another 2 minutes. Turn off the heat and pour 1 cup of the broth into a mixing bowl, add the miso paste to the bowl, and whisk until smooth. Return broth to the pot, stir, and add nama shoyu to taste.

HEARTY CHILI

Servings: 6

2 tablespoons extra-virgin olive oil

½ large onion, finely chopped

2 garlic cloves, minced

1 large carrot, peeled and diced

1 celery stalk, diced

½ green bell pepper, stemmed, seeded, and diced

1 cup corn kernels

1 teaspoon chili powder

1 teaspoon cumin

½ teaspoon ground chipotle

½ teaspoon cayenne pepper

1 teaspoon smoked paprika

12 fresh tomatoes, cored and pureed in blender

2 cups vegetable broth (see below) or water

2 cups cooked black beans

2 cups cooked kidney beans

3 tablespoons Raw Ketchup (page 145)

1 zucchini, diced

In a medium soup pot, sauté the onion and garlic for 2 minutes in olive oil over medium heat. Add the carrot, celery, green pepper, corn, chili powder, cumin, chipotle, cayenne, and smoked paprika, and cook until softened. Add the tomatoes, broth, black beans, kidney beans, and Raw Ketchup, increase the heat to high, bring the soup to a boil, then lower the heat and simmer for 50 minutes. Add the zucchini and simmer for another 10 minutes. Allow to stand for at least 15 minutes before serving.

VEGETABLE BROTH

Makes 3 quarts

   3 quarts filtered water
   4 zucchini, coarsely chopped
   2 carrots, peeled and chopped
   1 onion, coarsely chopped
   1 pound string beans
   3 celery stalks, coarsely chopped
   2 tomatoes, cored and coarsely chopped
   1 bunch fresh herbs (such as parsley, thyme, bay, or tarragon) tied
      up with twine
   Salt or yellow miso, to taste (optional)

Combine water, zucchini, carrots, onion, beans, celery, tomatoes, and herbs in a stockpot. Bring to a boil over high heat. Lower the heat, cover, and simmer for about 30 minutes. Remove herbs. Strain vegetables to use liquid as a broth, or add salt and puree in a blender to serve as a soup.

9
FREQUENTLY ASKED QUESTIONS

I love meeting people when I'm handing out samples of Brad's Raw products in stores. I love to see their curiosity about raw foods, I love explaining why eating raw food is so good for them, and I love hearing them talk about getting healthier and making smart choices about what to purchase and prepare for their families.

I tend to hear the same questions from both newbies and experienced raw foodies, so I've compiled the most common questions in this chapter. I hope you find the answers helpful.

What is a balanced raw food diet?

A daily menu should consist of a healthy blend of leafy green vegetables containing chlorophyll (such as kale, collards, spinach), fruits (such as melons, apples, oranges, mangoes), and fatty foods with protein (avocados, nuts, seeds, coconut).

The reasons for this are brilliantly simple: Foods with chlorophyll act as structural building blocks for the body because chlorophyll is similar to hemoglobin, which is the oxygen-binding substance in your blood. This similarity makes it easy for your body to assimilate chlorophyll. Fruits have sugars that fuel your body's need for energy. Fats and oils help keep the body's digestive system lubricated, your skin supple, and your brain functioning (yes, you really and truly do need good polyunsaturated fats for your brain to work properly!).

With the meal plans and recipes in this book, you can enjoy different fruits and vegetables every day. You'll never get bored!

Take a look at the lists of nutrient-dense foods in chapter 7. Very few fruits and vegetables are deficient in nutrients; all of them will provide you with delicious flavors and textures.

You want to have a rainbow of colors on your plate or in your bowl at every meal. Use the rainbow as your cheat sheet throughout the day. If you had something green for breakfast, make sure there are different colors on your plate later in the day. If you have carrot juice for a snack, munch on a red bell pepper pâté with your dinner.

Are raw food recipes complicated?

Not at all! My team and I worked on the recipes in chapter 8 for months to give you a delicious and foolproof arsenal throughout the plan. We particularly concentrated on maximum nutrition and variety so you can stay excited and satisfied about eating this way.

You might look at them at first and think, no way! But once you see how absolutely basic they are, there's really nothing to worry about. Like all recipes, whether raw or cooked, there are both simple and complicated versions. It's all about finding which ones you like and which ones make you feel comfortable. Nearly all the recipes are tailored to beginners and provide the proper nutrient density your body needs.

Most of the recipes require no special tools—only a blender or food processor. I did provide a short section on dehydrated recipes, because they are so much fun to make and so dear to my heart. You may even become inspired enough to purchase a dehydrator once you realize how much fun it is to use and what a simple yet incredible machine it is.

Is it going to be harder or more time consuming for me to prepare raw meals?

With just a little practice, anyone can make scrumptious raw food meals—believe me, I'm talking from experience. When I started with raw, all I knew how to do was turn on a blender and chop up vegetables. But half the fun for me was learning how to experiment with different ingredients.

There is always a learning curve when it comes to trying something new and getting into the rhythm of a new routine. If you have basic cooking skills, then you'll need to learn only a few new techniques, and once you master them (which is a very quick process), you will discover that you're likely to spend less time in the kitchen than you did before. You won't be bending over a hot oven, that's for sure!

One of the biggest differences between raw and cooked foods is that raw takes a bit more planning ahead. When you are making smoothies, juices, soups, and salads, prep time will be ultra-simple and quick, but sprouting or soaking ingredients, such as nuts, takes a little advance planning and some extra time.

Once you're comfortable with your new routine, it will be easier to try new, slightly more complicated recipes. Like anything, getting going takes a little practice, but pretty soon your training wheels will come off!

What should I know when I'm food shopping for my raw food meals?

These are my favorite shopping tips:

- Each week of the 8-week plan, look at the meal plans in part 2, then make a master grocery list with the following categories: produce, nuts and seeds, superfoods, spices, herbs, and dried fruits. Produce tends to be the bulk of what I purchase each week, and sometimes I shop for fresh produce several times a week, depending on my travel schedule. I pick up fresh herbs when I get my produce, as they're in the same area of the store.

  I always buy my nuts, seeds, spices, superfoods, and dried fruits in bulk, as it's much cheaper. When you get home, transfer them to labeled glass jars so you know what you have. Buy larger quantities of the nuts you tend to use the most, such as walnuts and almonds. You'll go through them quickly, especially if you make fresh nut milk.

- Go right to the produce department and load up your cart. Then you'll be less tempted to go for the packaged foods in the center aisles.

- Never shop when you're hungry, or with hungry children! That's when it's super easy to pick up something you don't really want, just to take the edge off your appetite.

- Look at store circulars before you get to the store, as different fruits and vegetables will go on sale each week.

- Support your local farmers! Buy local and buy seasonal at your community farmers' market. Local farmers tend to have much better pricing, especially if you become a regular shopper at their stand. Ask if their produce is organic, and if you see something new or unfamiliar, ask about it and how to prepare it. Most farmers sell their food at these markets because they love what they're doing—they're not just out to make a profit—and they're almost always happy to talk to you about growing things and food prep and what's especially delicious that week.

- Join a CSA (community supported agriculture) group in your area. It's one of the best ways to get fresh, local produce. Most CSAs will allow you to purchase a half share or full share, depending on your needs and the size of your family, and you'll have beautiful and local greens and vegetables waiting for you each week.

- Try to buy organic whenever you can. Here is the Environmental Working Group's Dirty Dozen Plus (produce with the highest contamination of pesticides) and Clean Fifteen (the lowest in pesticides). If you are on a budget, try to buy organic at least for the Dirty Dozen Plus foods.

WHAT TO BUY ORGANIC ACCORDING TO THE ENVIRONMENTAL WORKING GROUP

Dirty Dozen Plus	Clean Fifteen
Apples	Onions
Celery	Sweet corn
Sweet bell peppers	Pineapples

Peaches	Avocado
Strawberries	Cabbage
Nectarines (imported)	Sweet peas
Grapes	Asparagus
Spinach	Mangoes
Lettuce	Eggplant
Cucumbers	Kiwi
Blueberries (domestic)	Cantaloupe (domestic)
Potatoes	Sweet potatoes
Green beans*	Grapefruit
Kale*	Watermelon
	Mushrooms

*May contain pesticide residues of special concern.

Copyright © Environmental Working Group, www.ewg.org.

What are some of your favorite tips for fitting food preparation into a busy schedule?

Try to prepare as much as possible ahead of time. Make a large raw meal that you can eat throughout the week, like a raw lasagna.

When I first went raw I ate a lot of prepared salads. I did my shopping, washed all the veggies, cut them up, put them in containers, and I was good to go for days. I had no stress and no worry about any of my meals because they were all waiting for me, and it made me much less likely to veer off the plan because I knew the food was already prepared. I got into the habit of doing all my dehydrating for my snacks for the week every Sunday.

It's a breeze to simply grab an individually portioned meal or snack as you head to work, school, to pick up the kids, to work out, or to run errands. I still make at least three or four salads on Sunday and store them in the fridge. I always keep the dressing separate so nothing gets soggy. (You know how I love my crunch!) I often carried a bottle of raw, unfiltered apple cider vinegar in the truck with me and used that on all my salads. It helped with weight loss and has other great health benefits as well.

You can also make big batches of juice; it will stay fresh and delicious for about three days as long as you store it in tightly sealed containers in the fridge.

Having apples, bananas, nuts, carrots, celery, and cucumbers on hand will make it easy to be prepared when you're in the mood for a snack.

How do I stay raw when I have a family that still wants (and expects) to eat our old diet?

Being faced with the temptation of your old way of eating, with the sights and smells of the food you're used to and that you love, can certainly be a challenge, but having to prepare and sit through cooked meals and deal with leftovers when you have a family adds an additional layer of temptation. This is where a bit of mental preparation ahead of time has its advantages.

I've found that it really helps to keep a food journal. Some people prefer to write down what they ate after eating, but you may want to try writing down what you are about to eat, and possibly describing the process you took to prepare the meal. Visualizing your meal this way can make you appreciate it more, and pre-satisfy your senses! Buy a blank book you'll enjoy using and keep it handy in the kitchen, or try using an app if you're so inclined.

Try eating a small meal of your own before preparing food for your family. Make a large pitcher of green smoothies so you can sip one when you are in preparation mode. If you're in the mood for something sweet, keep a bowl of fruit on the kitchen counter, or if you're in the mood for something savory, have kale chips or something salty and crunchy on hand so you can satisfy your taste buds.

Keep in mind, too, that the cleanse portion of my 8-week plan lasts for only four weeks. Then you will transition to an 80 percent raw and 20 percent cooked eating plan that is easy to follow. By that time you'll be feeling so good that a lot of the cravings you've feared will no longer plague you.

How do you help your family eat in a healthier way when you're following a raw plan?

Give them a small portion of what you're eating. If they balk at what's on their plates, remember the basic principle of going raw, which is to add more to, not take away from. Simply make the regular meals they are accustomed to, but add a lot more raw to your plate and a little bit more raw to theirs. Don't push it, but I've yet to see a family not enjoy a fantastic salad with a raw salad dressing. Kids, especially, love dips and dressings, so simply put them on the table and let them try them without nagging. If they're not interested, enjoy more for yourself.

Also, just as you're taking on a new challenge by changing your diet, it is also an excellent opportunity to challenge your family to try raw meals. Who knows—they just might like them!

Most of all, make it fun. Show your children all the amazing new foods you're trying. Even very small children can push the button on a blender and watch the smoothies get blended—and you know that a child who helps out in the kitchen is a child who's much more likely to want to try the results. Ask your kids to help you make raw desserts, especially something they'll love, like Mayan Chocolate Truffles (page 180).

I'll bet that when they see how good you look and how much better you feel and how much weight you are losing, your loved ones will come around to your new way of eating and want to try it, too.

ERIN'S STORY: RAISING A RAW FAMILY

My name is Erin Sojourner Agostinelli and I live in Asheville, North Carolina. I have three children: my son, Jade Sequoia, and daughters, Miah Rose and Violetta.

Q. How did you become involved with raw foods?

A. I was living on a farm, and I was already into vegetables and really fresh food. I grew for restaurants and for the local Montessori school, for their salad bar. The kids would come out to my greenhouse and I would teach them about good things to eat.

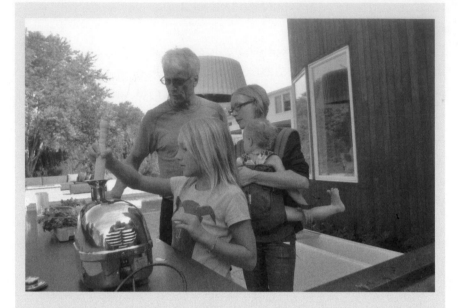

I started adding raw superfoods to my diet. These are foods with a high nutrient and phytochemical content that may provide health benefits, with very few negative properties such as saturated fat and artificial ingredients. I love spirulina and blue-green algae heavily sprinkled in nori salad/sprout wraps. I started making a spirulina dressing for all my salads, and my son loves it so much we even made it when we went out to eat at restaurants, packing the ingredients and mixing it fresh at the table before our salad arrived. The waiters always tasted it and were surprised at how incredibly delicious it was!

I soon had friends that were making raw lasagnas, and we'd get together and create recipes.

Q. When you're making meals, has it increased or decreased your meal prep time?
A. The kitchen is a place I end up hanging out a lot in anyway, but as far as prep time goes, I quickly learned how to rethink my week. It just takes a little bit of planning ahead, but once you get used to it, you don't really have to think about it much anymore. Meal planning is extremely easy. You soak all of your seeds; you can even dehydrate one day a week and place the results in your freezer, just as you'd do with cooked food.

Q. Do your children like to be involved when you're preparing meals or buying food?

A. I bring them into the kitchen as much as possible because that gets them involved in what's going on. Miah loves to make caramel corn and caramel apples, so we're trying to come up with a way to make a raw caramel sauce. Or we'll get out the natural mineral water and the girls will get vanilla cream stevia and we'll make our own vanilla soda. They love it. I can't tell you how lovely it is to hear them say, "Mommy, this is like magic. How do you make this stuff that tastes better than what's in the stores?" And they really mean it!

Q. As your three children are different ages, how do you integrate raw? If they grow up from day one eating it, like your youngest daughter, it's what they know. But Jade and Miah go to school. They go to other kids' houses. They see commercials. They go to restaurants. How do you make that work in the real world?

A. It takes a little bit of transition and a willingness to be open and adaptable. Because I always served them nutritious and delicious food, my kids grew up loving fresh fruit and veggies, and they actually crave miso soup, broccoli, and seaweed. They've adjusted their taste buds to natural sugars so they're much less interested in the kind of candy or sweets you see at the candy counter or bakery. It's about finding some kind of fun substitution, something that makes sense to their peers. Like raw chocolate. It's super easy to make incredibly delicious raw chocolate truffles and then not have to worry about them eating junk sugar.

Q. That's terrific advice. And I assume that you already know that if you ban any kind of food, that automatically makes your kids want it more, right?

A. Absolutely. It's never about taking anything away, but building on to what you already give them. My son sometimes wants to try things out that other people are eating, but then he'll say, "Mom when I have a soda with my friends I like it at first and I want to drink it, but afterward I feel like crap."

Q. How do you deal with the inevitable comments that arise from other parents?

A. One time when Jade was eight he was invited to a pizza party, and he knew he could eat the pizza if he wanted to. But he said, "Mom, can you make me a soup and some chocolate bliss before I go?" So I did. Sure enough, some of the parents at the party said, "You don't let him eat pizza?" I explain that I've always given my kids the option to eat what they want in a social setting, but that they know that they can turn items down if they don't want to eat them. If I'm in another culture or place— or my kids are—and something is offered to us, I'm going to try it and so are they! I'm never going to shut that out. You still need to let life be livable and fun.

Q. What is the most common misperception about kids and families eating raw?

A. That eating raw is vegetable sticks and nothing else, and that kids won't get nourished. I sprout a lot. I'll sprout lentils, but I lightly steam them because it makes them easier for kids to digest, and I'll throw the sprouts over salads. We usually have one big salad a day, which is just a smorgasbord of all kinds of good stuff. We also do activated almond butters and walnut butters—this means that the nuts have been soaked to activate the enzymes. Everyone's worried about protein all the time, and some people may need more protein than others, but needing a lot of protein at every meal is definitely a nutritional myth.

Q. What about lunches at school?

A. One thing I ask my kids is, How many colors did you eat today? Getting color into the diet, some greens or reds or blues, is an all-important component to the health of their bodies. I sent Jade to school with lunch boxes packed with yummy things such as seaweed and goji berries, and his classmates were fascinated and always wanted to try things. Even his teachers asked for tastings.

Q. What would you advise moms who are reading this book?

A. It's just a matter of adding on healthier items, bit by bit, so you can gradually replace what isn't so healthy. If your kids see you eating wonderful, nutritious food, they will be less averse to trying it. You'd be amazed how open kids can be to new foods if you go slowly and give them a chance to experiment with their palate.

Q. And you don't advise going too gung ho with it, do you?
A. No, I don't. I think cold turkey for kids—or for anyone!—isn't a good idea. I also think that you can turn them off to something if you push them too much.

Q. Is there a single most important thing for parents to do?
A. There are two things. The first is switching to organic. People will tell me all of the time, I can't afford it. But I see eating organic as health insurance for my kids now. I tell parents to look for food that comes in its most natural form, with the least amount done to it. And try to eat in season as much as possible.

The second is never take anything away—just start adding something new and see what works. For example, if your children like to make juices, start adding ingredients such as apples, oranges, and spinach to give them that wonderful burst of micronutrients.

Q. And be sure to look for community, too.
A. Absolutely. The raw food world has exploded, in a great way. Meetup .com is a terrific resource for meeting like-minded eaters and cooks. And if there isn't one in your area already, start your own! In my group, we have potlucks, recipe sharing, and different speakers.

Do raw food recipes require special or expensive equipment?

Not at all! Although a food processor or a blender is useful, you do not need to spend a lot of money on expensive equipment or ingredients. Choose recipes that are within your means of time allowance and kitchen tools you already have.

The one tool that is an absolute must—and this is for all food preparation, whether raw or cooked—is a sharp knife. Try to buy the best knife you can afford. A paring knife is also handy. A dull knife not only makes cutting a tedious process, but it can be dangerous. Try several knives at a kitchen supply or hardware store if possible to find one that feels best in your hand.

In addition, some inexpensive tools that are great to have are a nut-milk bag; a spiralizer, which slices veggies into thin strips, making it look like pasta; and sprouting jars or glass mason jars.

A dehydrator is a wonderful piece of equipment (and I owe all of the success of Brad's Raw Foods to the trusty dehydrator that allowed me to make my first kale chips), but it is expensive and takes up a lot of space. That said, once you get deeper into loving raw, you will find that using a dehydrator will give you a tremendous amount of creativity in your cooking. One of the most heavenly scents I ever smelled was a batch of raw apple and maple granola dehydrating overnight. It smelled (and tasted) better than any pie I ever ate.

Lots of raw foodies talk about a Vitamix blender. Do I need to have one?

When you first start eating raw foods, any sturdy household blender will do. There are many top-rated, high-powered blenders, so scout around online for recommendations and price comparisons. As you become more experienced and more excited about raw foods, you may want to upgrade to a Vitamix. It is an expensive blender with many unique features, and it is basically indestructible. I've yet to meet anyone who regretted purchasing one, as they use it every day because it works so well and makes all their food prep so easy.

If you don't own a blender or Vitamix, and don't want to purchase one, you'll need to chop your food finely to expose vital nutrients and to make your food easier to digest. This is tedious and time consuming. It's much easier to consume a higher quantity of raw foods using a blender in your raw meal plan.

Do I need to own a juicer, too?

Juicing provides a terrific boost of easily accessible energy and beneficial nutrients. It's great to have access to a juicer, but it's not mandatory.

If you don't want to invest in a juicer, use your blender instead. Simply follow the juice recipe by blending all of your ingredients until smooth, then strain the pulp through a fine mesh strainer or a nut-milk bag (although that will be a little messy!). This will extract the fiber and give you the fresh juice just as your juicer would. You can save the pulp and add it to your smoothies or other recipes later in the day.

What's the difference between blending and juicing?

Both blending and juicing allow the vital nutrients and enzymes of the raw food you're processing to travel straight to your cells and become instant nourishment.

As always, you want to consume everything in moderation. How many greens have you had, how many veggies, and how many fruits? Try to ingest all the different colors of the rainbow over the course of your day. When you do, you'll be eating and drinking the balanced nutrients that you need.

When you juice, you are not consuming the pulp of the fruits or vegetables, so you will not get as full as you would if you were to eat the plants.

In addition, if you drink only fruit juice, you will be drinking a lot of natural sugars. Bear in mind that large quantities of even the good kind of sugars will cause an insulin spike. That's why I think it's best to blend fruit and veggies together.

I often explain it this way to juicing newbies: If you have been eating an unhealthy diet and switch from breakfast muffins and bagels to juices made mostly from fruit, this will be better for you but still not optimal. Gradually adjust your proportions so that a primarily fruit-based juice becomes a primarily vegetable-based one, and you won't have to worry about insulin spikes after you drink it.

It is also very easy to underestimate how much sugar and calories you are drinking rather than eating—and I think this is one of the reason why people put on a lot of weight and can't figure out why; they're not counting the calories in the foods that they drink! For this reason, you will notice in the recipes that I have included only three juices that are fruit only.

Blending, on the other hand, keeps all the nutrients and pulp intact. You'll be drinking all the fiber of whatever you've blended, which aids in the digestive process and makes you feel full. When I first started my raw food diet, green smoothies were what set me up for success. Because I started my day with a shot of greens and nutrients, eventually the only cravings I had for the rest of the day were for equally healthy and nutritious foods.

Do raw food recipes require special or expensive ingredients?

Hard-to-come-by or exotic ingredients can help make dishes unique, but are by no means mandatory. As far as having to buy expensive ingredients, the most important thing is to use the best quality fruits and vegetables you can find that can fit within your budget. Try to buy organic whenever possible. If you can, choose organic produce for fruits and veggies with a soft skin, as it is easier for pesticides to penetrate them (avocados and grapefruit, for instance, are less likely to be penetrated by pesticides than strawberries and grapes). See the list on pages 204–205 for more details.

Remember, choose the foods you want to prepare based on what you like to eat and what you feel comfortable with. This should always be a fun learning process and should never feel overwhelming.

How much does it cost to follow a raw food diet for a month?

Food costs depend on your daily caloric needs and tastes. If you like to eat simply with not much variety, your costs will be lower than someone who likes to try a lot of different things, or who exercises a lot every day, which increases caloric needs.

Your food costs also depend on what's available where you live, and what types of fruits and vegetables are easy to obtain. I live in the countryside in Pennsylvania, but often go into New York City for meetings. I always try to go to the large farmers' market in Union Square to see what's available and support the farmers, and I know the prices will be a lot higher than at home in Pennsylvania—but that's because everything costs more in New York City! Buying dry ingredients in bulk will lower costs and help you keep ingredients on hand for when you need them. When I first went raw there were times that I couldn't afford all organic vegetables. At the time, it was better for me to be eating any kind of vegetable than the old diet I was used to.

If you haven't been able to use all the fresh fruit and vegetables you've bought, a neat way to keep them from rotting is simply to puree them, freeze them in labeled, dated containers, and voilà—you've got instantly usable goodness for your future smoothies. Or make a batch of fresh juice and drink it throughout the day. This will not only give you something wonderful to drink, but it will also prevent any waste of food or money—and it'll encourage you to drink something healthy!

When I start going raw, how will I feel?
When you switch to a raw food diet, you are likely going to be making a major change in the way you have been eating for years, if not your lifetime. So your body might be a bit puzzled at first, and it's going to react!

I don't recommend that anyone go cold turkey from cooked to raw as I did, and I've already described how I reacted. Gradually easing into raw should prevent many of the withdrawal symptoms I outlined in the introduction.

While it was very hard for me to get through the first few days, I knew what I was experiencing was totally normal, and that I just had to hang in there because the pot of gold would be waiting for me at the end of the detox rainbow.

What are typical detox symptoms?

I think it's always good to be prepared for what might happen, and then be pleasantly surprised if the bad things you expect don't happen. In other words, I am listing every possible reaction you might have, so don't let the possibility of these symptoms scare you off. You might experience all of the symptoms I had, one or two of them, or none at all.

Everyone's body reacts differently, depending on your age, physical condition, and what kind of diet you've been used to eating. I was eating a ton of junk and processed foods, and I didn't consider it a good day unless there was meat on my plate, so I had a lot of detoxing and cleansing to go through.

Detox symptoms can include headaches, bloating, stomachaches, skin breakouts, cravings for certain foods, restless sleeping, constipation, loose stools, fatigue, irritability, general achiness, and congestion. Some people will feel, as I did, that they have the flu.

On the brighter side, some of the good symptoms you will feel afterward are deeper and more powerful breathing, weight loss, bowel regularity, clearer skin, mental clarity, more restful sleep, and increased energy.

The best thing that happened to me was an improved sleeping pattern. When I wasn't on a raw food diet, I always struggled with sleep. Now I wake up each day feeling rested and energized. I know it's a big reason I have been so successful in my business. I have a clear mind each day to make big decisions for my company.

You might want to try to schedule your transition to raw for a time when you know your stress will be as minimal as possible and your schedule fairly flexible. Starting the program when you're traveling or when you're about to embark on a huge new project at work can make it harder to follow.

If you feel fatigued, get as much rest as possible. Drinking water will aid in flushing out the toxins more quickly, as well as make you feel full.

If I do have withdrawal symptoms, when will they go away?

Most people who've gone through this kind of cleanse have told me that their initial symptoms lasted from two to seven days, and occasionally lasted longer than fourteen days.

The duration and intensity of your symptoms will depend on what kind of diet you had been eating prior to starting the cleanse. Expect that your energy might be subpar for a week or two. But this fatigue will soon be followed by such a burst of energy that all the previous symptoms will quickly be forgotten. That's when you'll know that the discomfort was your body's way of telling you it had been long overdue for a good cleanse!

What if these symptoms don't go away after fourteen days?

As always, use your best judgment. Always consult your physician before embarking on any diet change or detox process, especially if you take certain medications (blood thinners, for example, preclude you from eating certain veggies that contain vitamin K). Listen to your body and follow intuition. If your symptoms concern you, speak to your physician. Periods of particularly intense stress might exacerbate your symptoms, too. You may want to get a blood test before starting the plan to see if you have any medical issues you might not have been aware of.

Will I feel full and satisfied during the Simply Raw portion of the plan?

Absolutely! Juices are very satisfying to the palate and the stomach—they are loaded with tasty nutrients. Smoothies are satisfying, too, because they have the pulp and fiber that help you feel full. In addition, many raw food dinners are prepared with nuts and seeds, which provide protein and satisfaction.

What's most important to remember is that if you feel hungry you should eat. Always have fresh fruit and vegetables and something crunchy available for snacks. You can drink hot tea, especially green tea, which is packed with antioxidants. This will help you feel full. Drinking plenty of fresh, clean water will help you feel full, too.

Steak tartare and sushi are raw, so can I eat them?

My eight-week plan is a raw vegan diet. I do know, however, that some raw food people do eat some meat, fish, and/or dairy in a raw state and thrive on their eating plan. While I have found maximum benefits by following a raw vegan diet, each person is unique. I suggest you finish the first two phases and then when living the 80/20 diet, add on sushi or steak tartare if you want to as part of your 20 percent.

This is not to say, of course, that I never eat meat. You already know that I eat cooked meat on occasion and I consider it a treat. But I can emphatically state that I have basically lost my taste for the big slabs of steak I used to eat several times a week. I really do prefer my food raw now. I am a huge sushi lover, so my 20 percent is often fulfilled at my favorite sushi restaurant.

Why isn't milk considered a raw food?

Milk straight out of the cow is most certainly raw. But even though there are many proponents of raw milk, there are risks to drinking unpasteurized milk, particularly for the very young, the very old, pregnant women, and anyone with a compromised immune system.

I've found that totally restricting all dairy can be one of the reasons a lot of people find it hard to stay on a raw eating plan, so if you are a cheese lover and you tolerate dairy products well you can include cheeses as part of your 20 percent on my 80/20 plan and enjoy every bite. Just try to use organic dairy products, or those from non-BHG and antibiotic-free cows as much as possible. If you nosh on some cheese one night, follow it up the next morning with some great green juices to keep those nourishing enzymes flowing. And bear in mind that your 20 percent should not solely consist of dairy products. Like sweets, try to consider dairy as a treat.

Can I eat grains?

Yes, you can eat certain grains as long as they are sprouted.

You may have seen "sprouted grain" bread at the health food store. Sprouting grains—which means you soak and then germinate the grains as you would a seed—makes the grains easy to digest. Sprouting activates the food enzymes of the grains and increases their vitamin content, particularly the B vitamins, and increases other key nutrients such as folate and essential amino acids. Studies cited in the *Journal of Nutritional Science and Vitaminology* and the *Annals of Nutrition and Metabolism* have stated that there are health benefits associated with eating sprouted grains, such as resistance to diabetes, protection against fatty liver disease, a lower risk of cardiovascular events, and decreased blood pressure. This makes sprouted grains a valuable addition to your raw food diet. They make great snacks and can be consumed raw, in salads or wraps.

While sprouting is not mandatory when you go raw, it's easy and fun to do. If you have kids, involve them in the process. I've yet to see a child who doesn't thrill at the sight of newly sprouted grains and seeds, and it helps them understand how food grows. Plus, they're a lot more likely to actually eat something they grew themselves!

What are good alternatives to bread?

There are many ways to make raw "bread" or crackers using a food dehydrator, and you'll find recipes for them in chapter 8. If you don't have a dehydrator, look for raw breads and crackers in your local health food store. Many small raw food cafés will dehydrate their own bread and might be willing to sell it to you for takeout. It's fresh, delicious, and filling.

I like to use thick leaves of kale or collard greens as "wraps," and use large marinated portobello mushroom caps instead of slices of bread.

I see coconut oil used in a lot of raw food recipes. What are the benefits of coconut oil?

Coconut oil has many benefits, both inside the body and out. Because of its high fat content, applying raw coconut oil topically helps your skin retain moisture, keeping it smooth and hydrated (plus, you smell yummy!). It also has antimicrobial properties, which can help protect your skin from infection.

Many people have a misconception that coconut oil is bad for you because of its high saturated fat content. The fat in coconut oil contains something called medium-chain fatty acids, which are much more digestible than most other oils. Unlike other types of saturated fats, medium-chain fatty acid helps convert fat into energy, so it's not stored in the body. This is excellent news for the fit and active healthy eater—because it makes coconut oil one fat you can feel good about. Using coconut oil in your raw food meals will also give you a multitude of vitamins and minerals, including vitamin K, vitamin E, and iron. It also contains a fatty acid called lauric acid, which supports the immune system.

What are fermented foods and why are they good for you?

Fermented foods are those that have begun to be broken down by organic acids, bacteria, or yeast to promote the presence of beneficial microorganisms in our digestive tract. Some examples are tempeh (made from soybeans), sauerkraut, pickled foods, kimchi (made from cabbage or other vegetables), wine, vinegar, yogurt, and kombucha (made from mushrooms). Eating fermented foods helps restore beneficial bacteria in your stomach lining. They also help increase the presence of enzymes that our bodies need to properly digest and absorb nutrients from our food. Zesty Kimchi (page 140) and Coconut Yogurt (page 131) are some of my favorite foods, and I enjoy them quite often.

What if I don't like nuts or seeds?

That's okay—there are many other options! You can fill your diet with fresh greens, veggies, and fruits. Or try incorporating nuts and seeds into a pâté or use them in a sauce.

What if I have nut or other allergies?

If you have nut allergies, you should use sprouted grains, dark leafy greens, and legumes as your protein sources.

Can I drink coffee?

This is a tough one—I know how much people love their coffee. Caffeine does have some health benefits and coffee tastes so good, but if you drink a lot of coffee you already know that caffeine is, literally, a drug. You also know that going cold turkey off caffeine will make you feel cranky, and crummy.

Coffee has no place on a raw food cleanse, as it is roasted above 115°F and brewed with boiling water. It is also dehydrating, and it is especially important to keep your body as hydrated as possible while on a raw food cleanse.

My suggestion is to start weaning yourself off caffeine several weeks before you start the 8-week plan. Simply start by replacing one-fourth of your regular coffee blend with decaf. Drink that for a few days, then increase the proportion to one-half, then three-fourths, and then fully decaf. Decaf coffee contains a small amount of caffeine, so you should not have any withdrawal symptoms by the time you're drinking only decaf.

It might be hard for coffee lovers to believe, but ultimately, with a raw food diet, you will notice a huge increase in your energy and stamina. You may not even miss your morning coffee routine!

During the three phases, you'll find it helpful to keep other hot drinks, such as green tea, handy. Green tea contains small amounts of caffeine, so it will make you feel better if you're experiencing withdrawal symptoms. Flavorful and decaffeinated herb teas will tickle your taste buds, too.

Once you complete the Basic plan, you might be surprised to find that you've lost your taste for coffee. I never thought I could stop my four-cup-a-day-loaded-with-cream-and-sugar habit, but I did. I also never thought I wouldn't miss coffee at all, but I don't.

Can I drink tea?

You can drink tea on a raw food diet, though during a cleanse avoiding caffeine as much as possible is a good idea. Green, herbal, and white teas are plant based and undergo less processing than black teas, and no fermentation. They also have less caffeine than black teas.

One question I sometimes get asked is whether tea is "cooked" or not. Yes, technically speaking, the boiling point of water is 212°F. Nearly all tea boxes give recommended steeping times, usually 150°F for two to four minutes for green tea, and 180°F for four to six minutes for white tea, which isn't boiling but very hot. If you're out at a restaurant and want to drink tea, it will be brewed at the boiling point. (If you're worried, you can ask for the tea bag on the side, and add some cooler bottled water to the cup to bring down the temperature before adding the tea bag.)

That said, I don't know anyone in the raw food community who measures the temperature of their tea! We know that the healthy benefits of the antioxidants found in green and other teas made with boiling or nearly boiling water outweigh any negatives, such as the minuscule amount of digestive enzymes in the tea leaves or herbs that may or may not be destroyed by the "cooking" of the boiling water. You can't make hot tea without hot water!

There are so many delicious, refreshing, and nutritious herbal teas available that I'm sure you can find some you'll love. Drink it hot or make a huge pot and keep it in the fridge for iced tea. Try to stick to decaffeinated teas as much as possible. One of my favorite herbal teas is Spring Dragon Longevity Tea from Dragon Herbs. It contains gynostemma, made from the leaves of a climbing vine found in Asia, and tastes pure, sweet, and delicious.

Can I drink wine?

Believe it or not, wine is considered a raw food because it is fermented and not cooked (beer and distilled liquors, on the other hand, are not). In order to maximize the cleansing effect of your raw food diet, however, and to avoid taxing your liver function during this process, you should avoid drinking wine during the first 8 weeks.

After, you can drink wine moderately. Many studies have touted the benefits of a single glass of red wine daily, for those who like it. Try to look for organic wine that is sulfite free, as sulfites act as a preservative and have been linked to morning-after headaches. Buy the best quality wine you can afford, and savor it. Personally, I enjoy my red wine, and have found organic, sulfite-free wines.

Fruit has a lot of sugar. How much can I eat during the day?

Fruit is a fantastic alternative to junk sweets and candy that rot your teeth and inflate your waistline.

That said, you do need to keep an eye on your fruit consumption, whether whole or as juice. While fruit is nutritious and a good source of fiber, it also contains a lot of sugar. Dried fruit, in particular, is at the top of the concentrated sugar list. This makes it a great snack when you're craving something sweet, but you have to watch the quantity you consume.

For example, I love dates and you'll see them used in lots of recipes. One date contains approximately 22 grams of sugar and up to seventy calories, depending on its size. Because I love dates so much, I remain aware of my portion control. Using dates sparingly is a wonderful way to get a sweet treat and all that good fiber into your body. Try adding one or two to a green smoothie and enjoy its deliciousness.

Your best bet is to try to eat more vegetables than you do fruit. Look for veggies such as cucumbers, summer squash, butternut squash, and sweet potatoes that have a sweet edge to them.

I know I'm addicted to sugar and want to stop eating it. Will my cravings for sweets go away?

It might seem hard to believe at first, but the more raw food you consume and the longer you stay off processed sugar, the more you will lose your taste for the sweet stuff. It's almost as if you are resetting not just your metabolism but your taste buds.

As for my own cravings, I used to be an ice-cream-and-cookie-aholic. But here I am, six years after I first went raw, and I am rarely tempted by sweets anymore. That said, I know how people struggle with their sweets cravings. Be kind to yourself and recognize that the taste for sugar is a part of what makes us human! Be sure to have healthy alternatives on hand so that when the cravings strike, you know there is something to eat that is satisfying as well as good for you. Try eating fresh fruit, a few figs or dates, or a handful of raisins or cashews. Put some grapes in the freezer and suck on one until it has defrosted in your mouth—that's one of my favorite tricks.

What if I crave something warm to eat or drink?

Herbal tea, or decaffeinated tea, is a good bet. You might also want to buy a food thermometer; they're inexpensive and you can find them in the kitchen section of a supermarket or hardware store. If you have one, and you want to "heat up" raw foods, you'll be able to keep an eye on the temperature so that it doesn't exceed 115°F. Heat your food gradually, and do it only on the stove top, as it's impossible to keep track of the temperature during microwaving or in an oven.

Food warmed up in a dehydrator will still retain vital nutrients, and if you have a Vitamix, you can use it to heat up soups without comprising nutrient density. (Yes, it is a pretty amazing device!)

How do I navigate restaurant menus?

If you're watching your weight, it can be hard to eat out. If you're watching your weight and on a raw diet (especially if you're new to raw), it can be even harder. All of the sights and smells of the foods you may crave—especially that tempting bread basket and the little tub of butter!—can be hard to ignore. Here's what helps me get through restaurant meals:

- Have a salad, a piece of fruit, or a small raw meal before you go out. This will take the edge off your hunger. (This is also a good tip for anyone who's watching calories.)
- Look at the appetizer and salad section first. Chances are extremely high that you will find something delicious to eat. Ask if you can have an appetizer or salad made larger for your main course.
- See what kind of toppings or additional veggies might be available. For example, if the restaurant serves side dishes of cooked

veggies such as green beans or asparagus, ask for them to be added raw to your salad. Also ask for the dressing on the side, or ask for extra-virgin olive oil and vinegar and dress the salad yourself.

- Drinking plenty of water throughout your meal will help you feel full and satisfied.

- Since many restaurants now post their menus online, see if there are establishments in your area with selections that will give you a larger variety from which to choose. If you find local vegan or vegetarian restaurants, the chefs will usually be able to prepare raw dishes for you, so don't hesitate to ask for your server's advice and recommendations.

- If you have a smartphone or tablet, you can download a useful app called Happy Cow, which allows you to search for vegan and vegetarian restaurants in your area.

- If possible, try to avoid restaurants during the plan, so you won't be tempted—although, of course, you will be pretty proud of your stamina and determination when you turn down your favorite dishes! Once you're on the 80/20 plan, save your 20 percent for times when you know you're going to be eating out, so you can savor your meal without any guilt whatsoever.

What do I do if I have to go to business meetings or other events that involve eating out when I'm doing the cleanse, or when I want to stick to my raw diet?

As with making meals for your family or going over to Grandma's famous Sunday dinner, preparation is the key.

If your meeting is going to be held at a restaurant, call ahead of time and see if they can accommodate you rather than simply arriving and hoping for the best. Most restaurants can at the very least prepare you a simple vegetable or fruit salad.

If that's not possible or if the restaurant can't accommodate you (some chefs will not or cannot deviate from the set menu), try eating your own raw meal before you go to the meeting, and stick to ordering water or tea. If the meeting is held at an office, bring your own meal. Assuming that the meeting is about business rather than the food consumed, no one should mind your eating habits as long as they don't interrupt the focus of the meeting.

I know I continue to mention smoothies, but they really are amazingly helpful, especially for breakfast meetings, where the table can groan under the weight of bagels, doughnuts, pastries, and coffee. As you sit in your meeting discussing your weekly goals, you may find yourself taunted by a delicious blueberry muffin staring you in the face. Such temptation is hard to resist even when you tell yourself that eating a sugary and calorie-laden breakfast treat will only make you feel sluggish by lunchtime and want to crash a few hours later.

Instead, imagine sitting in that breakfast meeting with a quart-sized glass jar filled with a delicious green smoothie. You can sip on it the whole time, and it will fill you up right away. You will not feel hungry and you will not be tempted to eat the treats spread out in front of you.

I know many, many people who have been able to stick to their raw food plans solely because they brought green smoothies to business meetings, whether at breakfast or lunches. Yes, at first there might be teasing, but once you explain why you are eating a healthier diet, I can assure you the teasing will stop. In fact, I know of one worker who ended up getting her entire department hooked on green smoothies because she brought them to all her meetings. They saw how much weight she lost and how good she looked and felt, and wanted to do the same for themselves.

Be mindful about your eating, whether at work or at home. You know why you're doing this cleanse and you know how good the results are going to be. Keep that intention with you as you move through your daily tasks.

What do I say to people who don't understand the principles of eating raw, or mock what I'm doing?

I never had anyone mock me or tell me I was nuts, except for a handful of the good ol' boys from my construction days. Once they saw how much weight I lost and how vibrant and healthy I looked, they changed their tune. They wanted all the details of what I was eating and whether or not it would work for them.

Be confident in knowing that you are doing this for yourself, your health, and your longevity.

It can also be helpful to start or join a potluck group in your area, or find a Meetup group. I have an online educational support system, which you can find through my website, and it's a vital part of my day. I love the comments and questions that I get from members. We're all in it together—I find support for my own needs as well as give support to others who are going through the same transitions in their lives.

If I'm not trying to lose weight, what kinds of foods should I be eating?

If you are not trying to lose weight you'll need to determine what your daily caloric needs are, and then use a pocket calorie guide or app to help you figure out how to meet them. Higher caloric raw foods include nuts, seeds, avocados, coconuts, bananas, dried fruit, and cold-pressed oils.

If I follow an intense exercise routine, how can I make sure I'm getting enough calories?

Good for you for working out so hard! As you read in the entry above, you should have a clear idea of your daily caloric needs, and then factor in how many calories you burn during a workout session.

If you mainly do cardiovascular exercise such as running, see how hungry you get after a workout. You don't want to get so hungry that you find yourself craving an entire bag of nuts. Eat small meals during the day, which will keep your metabolism fired up and your blood sugar at an even level; this should prevent any intense hunger pangs.

Add more calorie-dense fruits and vegetables, such as avocado and ba-nanas. You don't want to lose weight too quickly.

If you weight train, you may want to increase the amount of protein-rich vegetables, nuts, and seeds you're eating. You also will want to do some research about superfoods and raw/vegan protein powders that can be good supplements to your diet.

Is there any age limit to starting a raw diet?

Absolutely not! Unless they have a medical condition that mandates a specific diet or are under direct supervision by a physician for a preex-isting condition, people of all ages can follow a raw diet with complete success.

If you're older than fifty or so, bear in mind that the detox process during your cleanse may be a little more intense than it would be for someone in their twenties; after all, you've had more time to store up tox-ins in your body. During this time, drinking plenty of water and resting are very important. You might also want to try to sweat, if you have the energy to work out, as I did, because it helped me tremendously.

Listen to your body. Be mindful of the changes you're experiencing, and think of them as totally normal and all part of the process. They are temporary.

In fact, many women who are perimenopausal or menopausal often see a decrease in their symptoms during a raw diet cleanse. Treating your body well and giving it the optimum nutrition it craves can help allow your body to reset itself as you go through changes.

Do I need to adjust my raw diet when I'm menstruating?

You might find that a raw diet alleviates some of your symptoms—especially your intense cravings for sugar, if you get them—because you'll be consuming more nutrients and hormone-balancing foods.

The best ways to combat PMS are to include foods that are high in vitamin B_6, such as bananas, to help fight breast tenderness, depression, and anxiety. Avoiding alcohol and caffeine will help alleviate the ir-ritability factor, as well as breast tenderness and swelling. Magnesium-rich foods such as spinach will help control mood swings and bloating.

Cutting back on processed sugars will help control the fluctuation in glucose levels. And be sure to get enough calcium and Vitamin D from green leafy vegetables and other sources; women who have a high intake of these two nutrients tend to feel less severe PMS symptoms. Or so my female friends tell me.

If, however, you are already at a low body weight and have lost more weight on a raw diet, you should see your gynecologist if your periods become erratic or stop altogether. A woman's body must have a certain percentage of fat for menstruation to occur, and extreme weight loss or nutritional deficiencies (which you will not have on the raw food plan in this book) can throw a woman's cycle off-kilter. Make sure to increase your caloric intake, and talk to your doctor about an ideal healthy weight for your body.

If I am eating a raw diet, do I need to take vitamin and/or mineral supplements?

If you follow a 100 percent raw food diet; eat only organic food; regularly consume fermented foods that provide thriving, viable bacteria for a healthy intestinal tract; and ensure that your diet is completely balanced and filled with nutritious items such as sprouts and superfoods, you will likely not need supplements.

This is a perfect world scenario, however, and we live in the real world. I know how hard it can be to eat like this every single day, because we all lead busy lives, have families, and work in a fast-paced society where demands are constantly placed on our time and energy. It's hard to be able to source exactly where every single thing you eat is coming from.

I do not take any vitamin or mineral supplements, but I incorporate different superfoods and nutritious foods into my diet. I drink a lot of green juice and smoothies every single day and always feel very energized and nourished.

That said, everyone's needs are different. You need to take care of your own body. Taking a top-quality once-daily vitamin and mineral supplement is not a bad idea. It certainly can't hurt you.

Make sure you have a thorough blood workup at your next

physical—or sooner if you're feeling run-down or stressed—and have your vitamin and mineral levels checked. Discuss your needs and options with your physician or health care practitioner.

Most of all, never self-diagnose! It is easy to be swayed by the advice of someone working in the supplement department of a health food store or to read information online, but in truth most Americans eat vitamin-and-mineral-fortified foods every day (even if they aren't particularly inherently nutritious), and true deficiencies are rare. Some water-soluble vitamins, such as vitamins C and B complex, are not stored in your body and need to be replaced regularly. Other vitamins, such as A, D, E, and K, are fat soluble, and excess amounts are stored in your liver. Forever. Taking ultra-high doses of these vitamins can be dangerous to your health.

Take a good look at a daily vitamin-mineral supplement. The RDA, or recommended daily allowance, is probably lower than you think it is. Taking more than the recommended dose doesn't mean you will get more punch from your vitamins. Your body can process only what it truly needs, and then either excretes or stores the excess. In other words, you don't need to pay for vitamins or minerals you don't really need (it will give you very expensive urine and not much else), and you don't want to put your health at risk by taking enormous quantities of supplements, either.

Bear in mind, too, that vitamin and mineral supplements are not energy sources. They do not contain calories, and therefore can never provide true energy that fuels your body. Nor should you take supplements as a quick fix for weight loss or because you think that will be enough to replace nutrients you might not be eating in the day.

Herbal supplements can be helpful for certain medical conditions, but they can also be dangerous drugs with potent side effects. Don't fall for hype or uninformed opinions. Saying something is "all natural" is a catchall phrase that is basically meaningless (after all, arsenic and snake venom are all natural, but they'll kill you in a hurry!).

As with vitamins and minerals, never self-diagnose. Consult a certified herbalist or holistic health care practitioner if you're interested in herbal treatments to go along with your raw food plan. For more information and research on this topic, visit www.dragonherbs.com. Ron Teeguarden is very knowledgeable and is recognized as one of the foremost herbalists in America. Also refer to the resources at the back of this book.

Be sure to continue to eat a healthy, balanced, and nutrient-rich diet and use supplements only after a thorough discussion with your physician or health care practitioner. I know what has worked so well for me, but your own needs might be completely different.

Should I take a probiotic or digestive enzyme?

Probiotics are supplements containing the healthy flora that lives in our intestines and is responsible for a healthy gut and the normal processing of food. Many factors can upset this bacteria balance, most notably antibiotics (they kill the good bacteria along with the bad bacteria), a lot of sugar in your diet, and stress.

Regular use of probiotics can help combat bad bacteria and yeast that grows in an imbalanced digestive tract. They can also aid in diminishing symptoms such as gas, bloating, and constipation, and can help if you have irritable bowel syndrome, and/or impaired immunity.

There are many probiotics out on the market, and it is important to choose the right one. Look for one with an enteric coating, which is designed to withstand the passage through your stomach acid and get into your intestines, where it can do its work. Otherwise, you will be wasting your money and get none of the benefits of the probiotic pill.

Once your lifestyle and diet habits have been adjusted, you can stop taking the probiotic. If your digestive symptoms return, you might want to start taking the probiotics again.

If you are experiencing a lot of gas and/or bloating, you should consider taking digestive enzymes. These help break down and digest food more efficiently, and as a result will aid your cleanse and detox process. I do take digestive enzymes as needed.

What happens if I give in to a craving during the plan? Do I need to start over from the beginning?

Please do not beat yourself up about it! If you fall off the plan for one meal or one day, so be it. There is no reason whatsoever to be ashamed or guilty or angry. You're already on the road to health and wellness, and you should be commended for all the effort you've put into it already. My plan is not about deprivation, but about providing education and support so you can eat well, feel good, and continue living this healthy lifestyle.

If you happen to eat something cooked, I suggest you start fresh the next day with a green juice or smoothie and get yourself back on track.

At some point, of course, you'll need to ask yourself what triggered your going off the plan. Stress, frustration, or simply craving the foods you love the most can push you to grab for them when you don't mean to.

If you're really struggling—and I totally understand why that might happen—you might find it easier to seek the support of a nutritional coach. You can go to bradsrawfoods.com, where my health coaches and I are there, ready to support you through these lifestyle changes.

Your Food Diary

Keeping a food diary or journal is a good way to keep yourself accountable and motivated, and it's an effective tool to track the progress you've made and the successes you've accomplished.

BEFORE YOU START

What is your weight now?

What was your weight when you felt the best in your life?

What is your goal for the completion of the 8-week plan?

What is your ideal weight for long-term health?

List your three overall goals for completing this cleanse:

1.
2.
3.

WEEK 1: PHASE ONE—PREPARE

Date:

How many hours of sleep did you get last night?

Did you sleep consistently through the night?

How did you feel upon waking?

What foods did you "add in" today?

Did you eliminate anything from your diet?

How much water did you drink today?

What was your energy level like?

What did you crave?

Did you incorporate any movement today? If so, what?

Before bed, take time to write down three blessings or things you were thankful for from your day:

1.
2.
3.

(REPEAT THE ABOVE FOR EACH DAY OF WEEK 1.)

WEEK 2: PREPARE CONTINUES

Date:

How many hours of sleep did you get last night?

Did you sleep consistently through the night?

How did you feel upon waking?

What *two* foods did you "add in" today?

Did you eliminate anything from your diet?

How much water did you drink today?

What was your energy level like?

What did you crave?

Did you incorporate any movement today? If so, what?

Before bed, take time to write down three blessings or things you were thankful for from your day:

1.
2.
3.

(REPEAT THE ABOVE FOR EACH DAY OF WEEK 2.)

WEEK 3: PHASE TWO—SIMPLY RAW

Date:

How many hours of sleep did you get last night?

Did you sleep consistently throughout the night?

How did you feel upon waking?

List the raw foods you ate today:

List anything you ate today that was not raw. (Remember, the goal is 100 percent raw, but if you fall off one day, that's okay. Pick right back up from where you left off. Document it here.)

Did you have any cravings?

How much water did you drink today?

What detox symptoms did you experience today (if any)?

What was your energy level like?

Did you incorporate any movement today? If so, what?

Before bed, take time to write down three blessings or things you were thankful for from your day:

1.
2.
3.

(REPEAT THE ABOVE FOR EACH DAY OF WEEK 3.)

WEEK 4: PHASE TWO—SIMPLY RAW

Date:

How many hours of sleep did you get last night?

Did you sleep consistently throughout the night?

How did you feel upon waking?

List the raw foods you ate today:

List anything you ate today that was not raw. (Remember, the goal is 100 percent raw, but if you fall off one day, that's okay. Pick right back up from where you left off. Document it here.)

Did you have any cravings?

How much water did you drink today?

What detox symptoms did you experience today (if any)?

What improvements in your body are you starting to experience?

What was your energy level like?

Did you incorporate any movement today? If so, what?

Before bed, take time to write down three blessings or things you were thankful for from your day:

1.
2.
3.

(REPEAT THE ABOVE FOR EACH DAY OF WEEK 4.)

WEEK 5: PHASE TWO—SIMPLY RAW

Date:

How many hours of sleep did you get last night?

Did you sleep consistently throughout the night?

How did you feel upon waking?

List the raw foods you ate today:

List anything you ate today that was not raw. (Remember, the goal is 100 percent raw, but if you fall off one day, that's okay. Pick right back up from where you left off. Document it here.)

Did you have any cravings?

How much water did you drink today?

What detox symptoms did you experience today (if any)?

What new rituals/routines are you starting to incorporate into your daily life?

What was your energy level like?

Did you incorporate any movement today? If so, what?

Before bed, take time to write down three blessings or things you were thankful for from your day:

1.
2.
3.

(REPEAT THE ABOVE FOR EACH DAY OF WEEK 5.)

WEEK 6: PHASE TWO—SIMPLY RAW

Date:

How many hours of sleep did you get last night?

Did you sleep consistently throughout the night?

How did you feel upon waking?

List the raw foods you ate today:

List anything you ate today that was not raw. (Remember, the goal is 100 percent raw, but if you fall off one day, that's okay. Pick right back up from where you left off. Document it here.)

Did you have any cravings?

How much water did you drink today?

Have your detox symptoms diminished?

List three great feelings you are having today (mind, body, or spirit):

1.
2.
3.

Did you incorporate any movement today? If so, what?

Before bed, take time to write down three blessings or things you were thankful for from your day:

1.
2.
3.

(REPEAT THE ABOVE FOR EACH DAY OF WEEK 6.)

WEEK 7: PHASE THREE—LIVING IT!

Date:

How many hours of sleep did you get last night?

Did you sleep consistently throughout the night?

How did you feel upon waking?

List the raw foods you ate today:

Twenty percent of your food can be cooked. List the foods you ate today that were not raw:

Have your cravings subsided?

How much water did you drink today?

What stress busters or breathing techniques did you incorporate today?

Before bed, take time to write down three blessings or things you were thankful for from your day:

1.
2.
3.

(REPEAT THE ABOVE FOR EACH DAY OF WEEK 7.)

WEEK 8: PHASE THREE—LIVING IT!

Date:

How many hours of sleep did you get last night?

Did you sleep consistently throughout the night?

How did you feel upon waking?

List the raw foods you ate today:

Twenty percent of your food can be cooked. List the foods you ate today that were not raw:

Have your cravings subsided?

How much water did you drink today?

What stress busters or breathing techniques did you incorporate today?

Before bed, take time to write down three blessings or things you were thankful for from your day:

1.
2.
3.

(REPEAT THE ABOVE FOR EACH DAY OF WEEK 8.)

AFTER PHASE THREE—LIVING IT!

What is your weight now?

How much weight did you lose on the cleanse?

Besides weight loss, what other benefits happened to your body while on the cleanse?

Goals

Look back at your original goals. Did you complete them? Did you realign your goals at some point throughout the challenge?

List three new goals as you venture into your long-term 80/20 lifestyle:

1.
2.
3.

Congratulations on completing this journey!

Resources

KITCHEN GADGETS
Blenders

Vitamix
If you have the money, I suggest that you purchase a Vitamix. It is amazingly sturdy and versatile, and the more you use it, the more you will want to use it. One of the reasons I love the Vitamix is because you can make a whole blenderful of smoothies that will fit into a 32-ounce mason jar. That's enough smoothies to last you practically all week.

Go to www.vitamix.com.

NutriBullet
Although I haven't tried this blender myself, it comes highly recommended by superfood guru David Wolfe. It doesn't have the capacity or power of the Vitamix but is a much more affordable option.

Go to www.nutribullet.com.

Blendtec
This is another high-powered blender that I use at my office, and is similar to the Vitamix.

Go to www.blendtec.com.

Juicers

Green Star
This is an excellent household juicer, but it is expensive, so buy one only if you are certain you will be using it every day. Its twin gears do a terrific job and leave the pulp very dry.

Go to www.greenstar.com.

Champion
This juicer does not have a twin gear, so the pulp can come out a bit wet. I typically end up rejuicing the pulp a few times to get as much out of it as I possibly can. It is less expensive than the Green Star.

Go to www.championjuicer.com.

Breville
This is a centrifugal juicer that does a great job. I have one in my office. It works well for fruits and vegetables but is not the best for greens.

Go to www.brevilleusa.com.

Omega
This is a centrifugal juicer like the Breville and is quite affordable.

Go to www.omegajuicers.com.

Food Processors
My only recommendation is to use a big one, with a capacity of 9 cups or larger. In smaller models you'd have to halve many of the recipes, which creates additional work for you!

Dehydrators
You already know how I feel about dehydrators, but owning one is absolutely not a necessity. If you are interested in purchasing one, the Excalibur 9 Tray is a good option.

Go to www.excaliburdehydrator.com.

Sprouters
I have seen sprouters at raw food friends' houses, and they are awesome devices if you eat a lot of sprouts. They automatically water the sprouts so you

don't have to bother, but they are expensive, so I recommend one only if you plan to make sprouting a regular and substantial part of your raw food routine. Inexpensive sprouting jars that you water yourself can be found at health food stores.

Go to www.freshlifesprouter.com.

ONLINE RESOURCES

Information and Supplies

www.drfuhrman.com
Dr. Joel Fuhrman's site is an educational resource to help you lose weight naturally and prevent disease. You'll learn about his nutritional pyramid and gain access to his online library of resources.

www.davidkatzmd.com
This site promotes preventative medicine through nutrition.

www.mercola.com
Mercola.com is another terrific site for natural health information and access to natural health products.

www.longevitywarehouse.com
David Wolfe is one of the best-known raw food educators, and the Longevity Warehouse is a great resource for superfoods, super herbs, and organic foods.

www.jointhereboot.com
Follow Joe Cross, director of the documentary *Fat, Sick, and Nearly Dead,* as he journeys to bring health education to mainstream America. He is a resource for encouragement and inspiration.

www.hungryforchange.tv
A great resource for health information, where you will find amazing films to help educate and inspire you.

www.tcolincampbell.org
Learn more about the benefits of plant-based nutrition through the book *The China Study*, written by Dr. T. Colin Campbell and his colleagues.

www.michaelpollan.com
Michael Pollan has written several useful books. One of my favorites is *Food Rules*.

www.vimergy.com
Philip McCluskey is a motivational speaker and advocate for a healthy life. You can find his story on pages 38–39.

Food

www.therawfoodworld.com
This is the largest online raw food store in the United States, and has the best prices for items for your raw food kitchen. Website owner Matt Monarch also has an informative newsletter you can sign up for.

www.vitacost.com
You will find many things for your pantry on this website, which has very reasonable prices. This is where I go to stock up on items such as coconut oil, olive oils, raw food snacks, hemp seeds, goji berries, raw agave, lucuma powder, and more.

www.dragonherbs.com
Dragon Herbs is my go-to site for herbs, tonics, and teas, and informed details from a master herbalist. I love Ron Teeguarden's Longevity Tea. I also devour his goji berries, which are exceptionally flavorful.

www.nutstop.com
Buying nuts and seeds in bulk will cut your costs way down, and I love this site for its reasonable prices and large selection.

www.naturalzing.com
This is a well-run store that carries many different reputable brands.

www.abesmarket.com
Abe's carries many organic brands, natural body care products, and eco-friendly items.

Acknowledgments

I owe gratitude to many people who have helped me on my journey to raw and who helped me complete this book.

To my mom: I wish you were still here today, but I feel your love all around me. I know you are smiling down on me each day.

To my daughter, Eva: I think about you each and every day and love you very much. You have always been my guiding light.

To my sister, Pam Gruno: Your support has always proved invaluable to me. Your artistic eye and passion for this brand has ensured that we always stay true to our roots. Thank you for trying your best to keep me grounded. And to my brother-in-law, Richard Finch, thank you for your financial help when I first returned home. I realize what a chance you took with me. Your wood artisan skills are amazing—you have made the Chip Factory look fantastic.

To my dad, Bob Gruno: Thank you for having the confidence in me to put me in the positions you did within your company and allowing me to learn more about the corporate world.

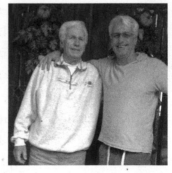

To Aunt Joyce and Uncle Brian: Thank you for welcoming me back to Bucks County with open arms!

To my business partner, Walt Gruger: Thank you for making your initial investment in Brad's Raw Foods and for taking a leap of faith and moving your family from Atlanta to Bucks County. We proved to be a dynamic duo!

To my father-in-law, Don Soberdash: I appreciate you allowing me to get my hands dirty and learn the hard lessons of running crews and dealing with different personalities. I have carried these lessons without me throughout my life.

Photo credit for my headshot goes to Shekinah Rae. Thank you for being a fantastic photographer and friend.

To Karen Moline: Thank you for taking the lead and for your impeccable writing skills on this project.

To Lauren Johnson: I appreciate your research and support of the book, which helped every step of the way.

Thank you to Alex Glass, my brilliant agent at Trident Media, who saw the future of raw and believed in my vision, and helped me every step of the way. Thanks also to his assistant, Michael Ferrante.

Thank you to my editor, the wondrous Sydny Miner, whose editorial expertise shaped every page of this book, and whose impeccable eye and instincts fine-tuned my initial concept and made this book soar.

And my thanks to all the people at Crown who helped make this book a reality, especially the publisher, Tina Constable; editor in chief, Mauro DiPreta; Sydny's invaluable assistant Anna Thompson; production editor Tricia Wygal; copyeditor Michelle Daniel; designer Lauren Dong; and cover designer Jess Morphew.

More than anyone, a very large and sustained thank-you to the indefatigable and irreplaceable Jaime Cahalan, whose support and belief in me were instrumental in making Brad's Raw what it is today. I would not be here without you, and this book would not exist without you, either!

And thank you to my entire staff at Brad's Raw Foods. I know times get crazy, but I appreciate each of you and the role you play within the company. Without your specific contributions, this wild journey would not be possible. I know the passion and commitment that each of you have is what makes this brand so successful. Much love.

Recipe Credits

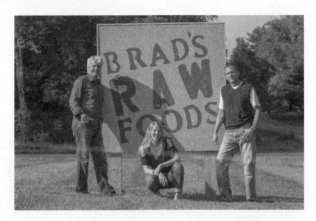

Recipes by Brad Gruno with the exception of the following:

JAMES BUSCH
Asian Coleslaw Salad
Deli Salad
Fennel Vinaigrette
Hearty Chili
Honey Mustard Dressing
Macadamia Alfredo Sauce
Marinara Sauce
Miso Happy Dressing
Pesto

JAIME CAHALAN
Baby Basil Dressing
Favorite Birthday Cake
Papaya Pudding
Raw Chocolate Chip Cookies
Tomato, Avocado, and Basil Salad

JOE CROSS
Mean Green Juice
Watermelon, Pineapple, and
Ginger Juice

ALEX MACK
Cucumber Juice
Pâté Rosa

PHILIP MCCLUSKEY
Cauliflower Popcorn
Pecan Spice Delight Cookies
Carrot Salad

EVA NORMAN
Green Seeds
Onion Bread

MICHELLE RACICOT AND ALEX MACK
Bloody Mary

MIAH ROSE
Brazil Nut Mylk Gone Wild!
Miah's Energy Balls
Kale with a Kick! Juice

MIAH ROSE AND ERIN SOJOURNER AGOSTINELLI
Zesty Flax Crackers

DANIELA TROIA
Burritos
Fennel and Orange Salad
Mango Mousse
Orange Vanilla Macaroons
Puttanesca Sauce
Zucchini Pizza

Index

ABOUT THE AUTHOR

Brad Gruno, Brad's Raw Foods

Brad's homemade snacks were met with a lot of enthusiasm from family and friends, and due to his entrepreneurial spirit, he quickly realized the commercial appeal they could have. He ran demos at local farmer's markets, and further praise validated the notion that his product had real potential. Soon, local health food stores and regional Whole Foods Markets began carrying Brad's Raw Chips. Since then, Brad's Raw Foods has been in a constant state of upward growth and expansion, and Brad's products are sold in specialty retailers and established grocers all throughout the country. His product line a now include Brad's Raw Chips & Crackers, Brad's Raw Leafy Kale, Brad's Raw 4 Paws, and his newest addition, Brad's Raw Onion Rings. Also, keep an eye out for further products such as raw energy bars, dips, snacks, and a new favorite: Brad's Raw Wine.

Though Brad's main job is to continue to oversee the success of Brad's Raw Foods, he also enjoys traveling and connecting with people all around the world in order to "spread the kale." He takes great pleasure in sharing his story and inspiring others to adopt healthier habits and lifestyles.

Raw food completely changed Brad's health and his life, and he hopes his products and company's mission will help do the same for you!

Visit **BRADSRAWFOODS.COM** to learn more about Brad, buy products online, to get health coaching, and much more!

BRADSRAWFOODS.COM f /BradsRawChips 🐦 @BradsRawFoods